Now, Men and Women Can Learn the Secrets to a Beautiful Body Through Weight Training . . .

The Hassle-Free Way to Get and Stay in Shape in Less Than Three Hours a Week!

LIFT FOR LIFE is the first complete guide for women and men who want to look better, feel better, and live better. All it takes is less than three hours a week in the privacy of your own home. Anyone can experience exciting, *dramatic* changes in their appearance, weight, strength, and how they *feel*.

Here is a myth-exploding book for all of those who thought that weight lifting was for *Pumping Iron macho*-men. Already, tens of thousands of working women, housewives, weekend tennis players, office workers, joggers, dieters, and businessmen are lifting for life, following this remarkable new system of exercise and body sculpting.

Whether you want to lose or gain weight, develop your back-hand or increase your endurance . . . LIFT FOR LIFE has the right exercise for you. Do you want broader shoulders, stronger wrists, leaner legs, a tighter mid-section? The programs to attain these goals—and dozens of others!—are clearly put forward in this fully illustrated guide, with dozens of illustrations and photographs by the co-creator of the best-selling *Art of Sensual Massage*.

LIFT FOR LIFE!

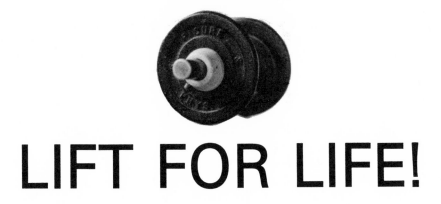

LIFT FOR LIFE!

A Personalized
Exercise Program For
Women and Men

for slimming, stronger
tennis, body sculpting,
and better health

by Vanessa Sing

Illustrated by Pedro Gonzalez

BOLDER BOOKS

NEW YORK

No way, no how, did this book materialize through the author's efforts alone. Thanks to everyone who helped to put it together, including our good-natured models: Adelia Fritts, Lisa Halbo, John Marshall, Karen Cotta, Alan Rinzler, our cover models, Robert and Jacqueline Argand, and our professional body builders Oscar Chung, and Dale Adrian.

And to those who went beyond the call of duty, special thanks: Brenton Beck, Evelyn Hsu, Pedro Gonzalez, Hal Hershey and Alan Rinzler.

Also, to Barbara Pascarella (for her invisible support): thanks, kiddo.

And especially to BILL REYNOLDS (for his highly visible support, advice, and generosity . . . and for restoring my faith in muscle mankind), without whom the book could not have happened: my warmest gratitude.

Copyright © 1977 by Vanessa Sing
Published by Bolder Books
a division of Hampstead Hall Press, Ltd.
10 East 40th Street
New York, N.Y. 10016
This book may not be reproduced in whole or in part by any
means without prior express permission of the publisher.

Library of Congress Catalog Card Number: 77-72262
ISBN 0-918282- 02-0

Cover design by Tony Lane
Book design by Hal Hershey
Photography by Robert Foothorap

Bolder Books
a division of Hampstead Hall Press, Ltd.

Distributed by Farrar, Straus & Giroux, Inc., 19 Union Square West, New York, N.Y., 10003

Printed in the USA.

Contents

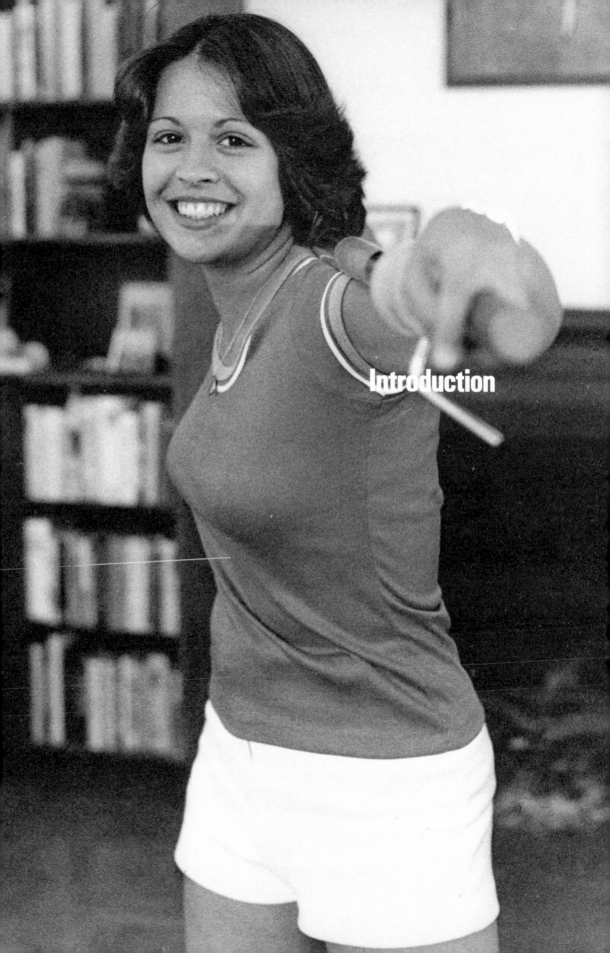

Introduction

All Aboard the Weight Train!

This book will get you started in what has in the past been considered a terribly exotic form of exercise: weight-training. The fact is that anyone of normal health can do weight-training. It doesn't take much gearing up to start, and you can benefit from the fruits of your weight-lifting labor very quickly — by feeling, looking, playing, and working better.

In the past when someone mentioned lifting weights, immediate images of muscle-bound idiot men would dance sugarplums in your head. Thanks to the recent interest in physical fitness and to body-conscious people's growing willingness to explore and experience the unknown, that is no longer the case. Now just about everyone realizes they can do it.

Weight-training means what it sounds like: you train your body with weights to become stronger and more efficient. The process is called *progressive resistance* training because you gradually increase your body's ability to deal with a greater amount of resistance (weight). Some of the exercises that are described later will be familiar to you, as they're often done without weights (e.g., sit-ups). But the reason this book recommends using weights for most exercises is that they are a very effective tool for working all the muscle groups of your body harder and better and for giving your body the shape you want.

Weight-training is a form of exercise that — when performed properly and with regularity — can joyously enhance your health, your strength, your performance in sports, and your mental outlook. In addition to priming you for any vigorous physical activity, it can concretely change your self-image — *outwardly* by redesigning your body's appearance, and *inwardly* by strengthening your concept of control over yourself and that thing you walk around in called your body.

Weight-training leads to faster results in terms of changing your body's tone and shape than exercising without weights. By carefully selecting exercises, you can isolate specific muscles or muscle groups, so that there are no wasted moments or movements if you wish to improve only certain areas. It is strongly suggested, however, that you first follow one of the general fitness programs at the beginning of Chapter 5. Then, as you become familiar with weight-training, you can try other programs or design one to suit your particular needs.

Weight-training should not be confused with the Olympic sport of weight-*lifting* or with another competitive sport known as power-lifting. (Both of these sports involve lifting as much poundage as possible, but differ in the types of lifts that competitors must complete.) "Bodybuilding" would be a good term to describe what this book is going to teach you to do, but that also connotes competition. Technically, body-building is an acknowledged sport in which men prepare their bodies with weight-training to compete on a stage (somewhat like a beauty contest). Actually, we'd all be a lot healthier if only we would assume the attitudes and some of the practices of body-builders. The unfortunate fact, as Veronica Geng wisely points out, is that ordinary people don't "build" their bodies — they just sort of accumulate them.[1]

Just sitting still for life can become a habit. But, like giving up smoking, many people have gotten it into their heads (and bodies) to stop trashing themselves – with nicotine, with too much alcohol, with junky diets . . . with inertia. Judging from the soaring sales of warm-up suits, fancy sneakers, and other athletic equipment, many former sedentaries have jumped that first hurdle and are now becoming doers.

Our bodies crave and need exercise. A fleshy, soggy, and saggy body speaks an unpleasant truth. Being out of shape probably means you look it. "Well, after work I'm too tired to exercise." Or, "After picking up after the kids all day, I'm too exhausted to exercise." These are typical excuses. But, especially if you've ever done any good exercising before, you know deep down that these excuses are nonsense. Good exercise stimulates. Far from being enervating, it revitalizes you and allows you to make better use of your time and energy. It can also help you live longer.

But Why Weight-Training?
It's easy for everyone to agree that all of us should, to some extent, incorporate an exercise program into our lives. But why weight-training? The best reason is that it can, when combined with a good cardiovascular activity (e.g., running, cycling, swimming), provide the best all-around exercise program, requiring less time but producing more dramatic results than any other form of exercise.

Because weight-training is based on progressive resistance, you design and perform workouts according to your own pace, physical size, ability, and personal goals. As the current Mr. Olympia (bodybuilding's most prestigious title) Franco Columbu sees it, "The real magic . . . is that it can be so completely tailored to you and the precise results that you want."[2]
When you first start swimming or playing tennis, you suddenly subject your entire body to all sorts of new stresses, rapid movement, and unfamiliar demands. With weight-training, however, you can begin with very light weights (as little as 1¼ lbs. in each hand), and you can choose the body parts you want to work. Consequently, you can break in your body very slowly – making weight-training a safe form of exercise. It also helps to prepare your body for the demands made on it by sports like running or tennis, as well as for everyday physical and emotional traumas.

There is a disadvantage to simply doing calisthenics, as weight-training instructor and expert Bill Reynolds points out. You have to possess a certain amount of strength before you can even begin, since you must use your entire body weight in doing the exercises. And the weight of your body also puts an absolute limit on the amount of work you can do, i.e., you cannot add weight and work harder – even if you want to and are capable of it. But with weight-training, you can start with 2½ lbs. total weight and work up to your heart's (and body's) desire. To give you an idea of what's humanly possible, the official world record for a squat hovers around 920 lbs. Champion Paul Anderson is rumored to have lifted 1,200!

Another important plus to weight-training – and an obvious one – is that this form of exercise can increase your strength to a degree and within an amount of time that other exercise programs simply cannot match. And you'll discover that your body responds very quickly in pleasing, cosmetic ways: you start to look better almost right away. Whether you're a woman or a man, things that used to flail about (like loose thighs and fatty upper arms) begin to tighten up and assume a more pleasing shape. Weight-training *literally* gets your body together.

In addition to prolonging your life, proper exercise has another salutory aspect: it can help prevent injuries, as well as rehabilitate body parts that have been weakened by injury or illness. Tennis great Billy Jean King now maintains that if she had only started weight-training earlier (she's a relative novice at it), she wouldn't have had the knee injuries that have plagued her. And Bill Reynolds loves to recount stories of body-builders who have been in horrendous car crashes and not only survived but quickly recovered, despite skeptical prognoses. The reason for this, claims Reynolds, is that these bodybuilders were in a superior state of general fitness before their accidents, and their incredible muscular development shielded them from more severe injury, or even death.

Another benefit of weight-training is that it usually helps people to sleep better. This doesn't mean that you should work out before going to bed (any exercise stimulates you and will keep you up for a while). Having a good workout during the day, though, will help convey to your body the message that it needs rest. As weight-training instructor Evelyn Hsu told me, "It definitely improves sleeping patterns. A lot of the time you can be mentally tired, but your body isn't. With weight-training, your body is able to catch up with your mind in terms of fatigue."

Also, because in weight-training you have to be very careful to go from maximum possible extension of the joint to the maximum contraction of the muscles that artic-ulate that joint, you tend to become more flexible. This counters a prevalent myth that weight-training makes its practitioners tight and muscle-bound. Hogwash!

Everyone's Got the Time
One amazing thing about weight-training, as opposed to other forms of exercise, is how quickly you can get results. And how little time you have to spend to achieve your goals. A beginner's and intermediate's program should consist of only three 45-minute workouts each week. That's a total of only 135 minutes of exercise a week.

You may be unable to perceive the changes in your body at first (just as you're the last person to see any weight loss or gain, simply because you're too used to being inside your own body). But friends and acquaintances will begin to notice improvements. Many people who are now fervent weight-trainers fondly remember how they first became aware of their own improvement through the eyes of others. "My, what nice shoulders!" is a frequent first comment from onlookers. What gets improved first, of course, depends on what program you follow and how diligently you adhere to it. But you can, especially at first, make great strides. Bill Reynolds maintains that it is not at all rare to have a strength gain of 50-100 percent in a matter of six weeks! And, as a sweet trick of Mother Nature, the weaker you are to start and the worse shape you're in, the more dramatic the first results will be. Thus, those who need the most motivation to continue get it.

Kicking Sand in the Face of Myths about Weight-Training

Only recently has weight-training been taken seriously as a form of exercise that a person of any size, sex, or intelligence can do. It's no accident that people who are supposedly vacant upstairs are called "dumbbells." And prejudicial expressions like how muscular people must be "muscle-bound between the ears" still exist.

The hero in the film *Rocky* says to his girlfriend, "My dad said, 'You weren't born with much brains, so you'd better use your body.'" And she replies something like, "That's funny. My mother told me exactly the opposite: 'You weren't born with much of a body, so you'd better learn to use your brains." Not long ago, everyone automatically saw this dichotomy between the mind and the body. People foolishly believed that if you were intelligent you wouldn't waste time exercising your body. Only your mind needed to be massaged and stimulated. And vice versa: if you were an athlete, you were a cretin . . . incapable of rational thought or artistic creation. Even among athletes there have been the usual myths about how weight-training makes people less flexible and restricts coordination. Nothing could be further from the truth. In fact, recent tests have shown that progressive resistance training improves athletic performance — helps people in various sports be quicker, looser, more coordinated, and certainly more powerful.

Another myth is that if you stop weight-training after you've been at it for a while, all your newly acquired muscle turns to fat. Again, untrue. The common-sense answer is that if you stop weight-training it will take about as long to get back into the dismal shape you once were in as it took to get out of it. In other words, if you were a mess and worked yourself into physical perfection in one year, it would take another year (of doing no training or exercise at all and reverting to your old diet) to return to where you were at the start.

How about your chances of becoming an Amazon freak? No such luck. Most people will never attain the degree of muscularity that bodybuilders display. What people forget or don't know is that those bodybuilders get that way via some very extreme methods. By following a moderate weight-training program and by eating normally, you simply cannot resemble those musclemen you see on the beach. Remember that bodybuilders live a life that revolves mainly around the art and science of bodybuilding. This may mean training three or four hours daily, eating incredible quantities of food, ingesting hundreds of pounds of food supplements, and taking anabolic steroids to build up muscle size. In other words, it takes a lot of work, food, will power, and sacrifice to become a big hunk.

This is not to say that you can't make great strides by following the programs given in this book, but unless you drastically change your diet (to either gain or lose weight) and train much more than the suggested 45 minutes three times a week, you'll remain basically recognizable — only much firmer and with better-defined musculature.

Not for Men Only: Women & Weight-Training

Myths about weight-training have particularly held women back from benefiting from its practice. But thanks to changing attitudes and some intrepid, pioneering women, thought and deed are being revolutionized concerning women and their rightful place in the locker room.

Swimming star Diane Nyad points out how recent studies explode common myths about weight-training, especially as they concern women:

According to Dr. Jack Wilmore, head of physical education at the University of Arizona, weight training will produce a great improvement in strength, with negligible increase in muscle mass. Wilmore reports that women will generally develop one-tenth the muscle mass of a man the same size doing the same weight program. Dr. Joan Ullyot, a California physician and marathon runner, contends that only one out of every 20 women shows significant increase in muscle mass because of a genetic potential to produce androgen.

Most women do not produce the hormonal secretions necessary for the formation of large, defined muscles. Just as estrogen in women spurs the development of the proper secondary sex characteristics, testosterone produces greater musculature in men. The overwhelming majority of women are not capable of developing enormous muscles, and need not worry about turning into Amazons.[3]

Billy Jean King frequently expresses her hope that other women will emulate those women athletes who have begun to take weight-training seriously. In her own words: "The social stigma that has prevented women from developing their bodies is evaporating as myths are replaced by facts." She reiterates that women simply can't develop bulky muscles from using weights in a normal program, since women don't have the right kinds of hormones. But, she says, "Women can get valuable strength and flexibility from working with weights — without the bulk."[4]

The fear that many women have of becoming masculine from weight-training is groundless. Physiologist Philip Rasch claims that in recent years most California beauty queens have trained with weights.[5] This makes perfect sense, since what actually happens to women who weight-train is that they become curvier and firmer. Apparently, back in the Fifties, Marilyn Monroe posed exercising with weights, and that got some novelty mileage for weight-training promoters at the time. And, as examples like Racquel Welch, Elke Sommer, and Ursula Andress (all rumored to weight-train) amply demonstrate, it's nearly impossible for women to become muscular in a lumpy, bulky sort of way.

Shirley Patterson, a 5'2", 112-lb. grandmother who has been lifting weights for about twenty years and who teaches 150 women at the North Hollywood Health Club, feels that most women have different goals than men.[6] Whereas men generally want to increase strength, women see weight-training as a way to condition the body — and incidentally to become stronger.

Dale Adrian, a bodybuilding champion who also teaches women weight-training, claims that although there were only a few hundred women who weight-trained three or four years ago, there are now about 10,000 in the United States. He attributes this to the fact that many of these women are under age twenty-five and young enough not to be "crushed by the old stereotypes in sports. Today women are much freer and more accepting of the idea that there is no such thing as a masculine or feminine sport."[7]

Other women are taking up weight-training to become stronger and more physically fit for certain kinds of jobs traditionally open only to men. With Equal Opportunity Employment mandates, women are now competing with men for jobs that require considerable strength. There are grueling physical examinations required for anyone who wishes to become a fire-fighter or police officer. Evelyn Hsu helped prepare women in Oakland, California, based on a program developed by Ann De Kervor, for passing the Oakland Police Department physical endurance test. Ironically, so much emphasis was placed on the physical aspect that many women who overcame that obstacle stumbled when it came to the written exam because they had put so much time, energy, and focus into the physical end of it.

There's almost a reverse jock revolution going on among women. It's a great conversation starter or stopper for a woman to announce she's running three miles a day *and* lifting weights. Men disbelieve; other women get very curious, especially if they like the way the weight-training woman looks.

Which brings up another stubborn myth about weight-training: that you gain weight. You may gain a few pounds simply because muscle weighs more than fat. But your measurements get smaller since you're tightening up. Evelyn Hsu has watched her students remain the same weight, yet lose two inches of thigh and an inch of waist. What happens is your body gets compact. If you do gain weight, you should realize that this means an addition of an aesthetic couple of pounds — as opposed to the ugly fat usually associated with weight gain.

If you're hung up on not weighing more than a certain amount, you should revise your thinking. After all, what really counts is how you like what you see in the mirror, not what your bathroom scale says. That's why it's suggested you check in with yourself during weight-training by looking carefully at your body in a mirror once every four to six weeks. You can also weigh and measure yourself regularly to keep track of your progress if you have certain goals to meet.

On the other hand, it's quite possible to lose weight, too. Weight-training is vigorous exercise; not only do you burn up a lot of calories, but it depresses your appetite. (I've found a good way to lose weight is to exercise at my normal dinner hour. This serves to destroy my appetite for at least an hour. And by that time it's too late to bother with cooking, so I end up skipping dinner. As long as I've had a good breakfast and lunch I function perfectly well.) Remember also that your metabolism (how fast your body burns up food) may increase a bit due to weight-training, and that might prevent weight gain, even with greater caloric intake.

That weight-training is becoming a more popular form of exercise for women is indisputable. Ask coaches in college weight rooms. Ask professional coaches or athletes. Ask owners of health spas and commercial gyms. There is no reason a woman should lose her feminity by lifting weights.

Within sports, more and more women athletes have started to weight-train. According to Sally Platkin Koslow, "It is now acceptable to be strong. A hippo of a lady wrestler is far from our ideal, but thinness . . . has ceased to be an end in itself. The same body freedom that churned throughout the recent sexual revolution now storms within the sports revolution."[8]

Just to name a few, Julie Anthony, Billy Jean King, Rosie Casals, Martina Navratilova, and Margaret Court have all discovered that weight-training adds power to their tennis game. Gymnastics instructor (and a member of the 1964 Olympic team) Muriel Grossfeld has developed a weight-training program for young gymnastics students (the attitude about whether gymnasts should train with weights has turned around quite a bit). Lucille Kyvallos, coach of a women's basketball team, especially encourages off-season weight-training to develop overall strength. Champion volleyball player Mary Jo Peppler has been lifting weights since 1967 and strongly believes that it's weight-training that has made the Japanese players as phenomenally good as they are. Olympic silver medalist Joan Lind maintains, "There isn't a decent woman rower in the world who doesn't treat weight-lifting seriously."[9] And Mickie King, championship American diver and coach, points out that not only does weight-training develop a diver's biceps and triceps, but it also, by trimming and toning the body in general, enhances the diver's appearance on the board.

For women in general, Diane Nyad comments, "All apprehensions about weight-lifting are disappearing. Women athletes are realizing that there is more to weight-training than bodybuilding. Weight-training increases flexibility and speed; it prevents injuries and rehabilitates them."[10]

Who's Fit to Weight-Train?
Weight-training is the perfect answer to greater fitness for all people who are busy and have little time to devote to exercise. Among other prime candidates are people who want to look and feel better, athletes who want to improve performance in a specific sport, anyone who depends on his or her appearance for professional purposes — many models and actors weight-train — and anyone who wishes to build strength in order to prevent injuries, to rehabilitate a weak body part, or to live longer and with more vitality. (Patients who require rehabilitation have long been given progressive resistance exercises to do under medical supervision; much of physical therapy is based on the same principle as weight-training.)

All kinds of people besides Arnold Schwarzenegger (the reigning king of bodybuilders) are currently weight-training. We've already mentioned a long list of women athletes. Examples of some of the better-known weight-trained male athletes could go on forever. Just to toss in a few names, there's Mark Spitz (remember him?), Bill Toomey (1968 Olympic decathlon champ), baseball players Joe Rudi and Joe Morgan, and O. J. Simpson.

The weight-training fever has even hit Hollywood. Nik Cohn reports in *New York* magazine that "a whole new breed of aficionados has emerged" under Schwarzenegger's rule. "Hollywood stars — Jack Nicholson, Warren Beatty, Jeff Bridges — flock to him for tuition; of late, the fever has spread east. Suddenly, at Elaine's, at Regine's, it seems that no man can pass as a truly Beautiful Person unless he works out."[11]

What Cohn neglects to mention is that Beautiful Women regard weight-training as an exotic "in-thing" as well. And who better to lead the pack than jet-setter designer Diane von Furstenburg? Chatter Box, in *Women's Wear Daily*, reports, "The sinewy 'Pumping Iron' look is pulling its weight among New York's Beautiful People. Diane von Furstenburg says she's been doing exercises to develop 'a little muscle' in her arms. 'I think it's the newest thing — very sexy, especially in thin women,' she says."

Heightening the fever, *Newsweek*'s March 7, 1977, issue showed a photo of Metropolitan Opera tenor Luciano Pavarotti pumping iron in a New York health club and quoted him as saying the weights "feel like a pillow in my hands."

Why Get Stronger?

There are many good reasons for increasing your strength. Jim Murray, author of *Weight Lifting*, provides some:

... Strength proves advantageous to everyone, including ... 'Mr. Average Man,' even though he be a white-collar worker. It is obvious that when athletes are equally skilled, those with more strength have an advantage. Also, when the workman is stronger than he needs to be, his everyday tasks prove easier to accomplish. Mr. Average will find strength an advantage when he is called upon to perform some unusual exertion, such as moving furniture for the wife during spring cleaning. If our Mr. Average were used to lifting a 75- to 100-pound barbell a few repetitions three times a week, he would be far less likely to bring on muscular strains moving a sofa than if his sole activity consisted of tottering from said sofa to the dinner table and back.[12]

As for women, to whom this book is very much addressed, being stronger has a definite psychological impact. Shirley Patterson says, "The immediate effects are a better contoured body, but the long-range effects are even more important. They (women) feel better, and besides, weight-lifting lets them prove to themselves that they are strong, vibrant, and very much a female in a sport that should have as many women as men."[13]

Being strong, as more and more women are discovering, contributes to a sense of confidence and control over their lives. Just as a lot of bodybuilders got into it because they were small and scrawny — underdogs — women have found that when they become physically stronger they think stronger about themselves, their capabilities, and their self-image.

Sally Platkin Koslow observes, " ... as more and more women rear against the concept that theirs is the intellectually weaker sex, they also question the equation of frailty and femininity." She quotes Beth Partridge, a Penn State hurdler and quarter-miler: "My body really doesn't desire to be a puddle."[14]

I suspect that most women who care about their vitality, longevity, and appearance would agree that they don't want to be a puddle, and that they don't want to muddle through life as wan and waif-like Ophelias, to be forever protected by macho lifeguard types.

You're Never Too Old ...

You can start weight-training at almost any age — from about twelve upwards. There's a feeling that children younger than that shouldn't do it since their bodies are still undergoing critical development and growth. As long as you don't have a severe physical problem or condition (rehabilitation should be medically supervised), you can weight-train to some extent. Often paraplegics, people in their eighties and beyond, and the blind can benefit from this form of exercise.

If, because of some physical condition, you have any doubts in your own mind whether you should weight-train or not, please consult your physician before starting any of the programs.

In my encounters in the weight-training world, I have seen people of all sizes and shapes in the act. And they all have stories to tell about older people — folks in their seventies and up, even centenarians — who weight-train. One of the best examples of a geriatric bodybuilder is Sigmund Klein, who for many years ran a famous health studio in New York. According to all accounts, Klein still trains although he's now over 80; and except for his skin texture (age causes loss of elasticity of skin), he has the body of a man in his twenties.

Many weight-trainers have been devotees since they were adolescents. Others take it up relatively late in life. Needless to add (but I'll add it anyhow), I've never seen a weight-trainer over sixty, say, who looked his or her age. When you think of growing old you think of a decayed, feeble body. Weight-training just doesn't allow that to happen to you.

Veronica Geng reported in an article she wrote on bodybuilding that the subjects of her research kept proudly asking, "How old do you think I am?"[15] Unlike athletes in other sports, where being thirty years old may mean "over the hill," bodybuilders tend to peak later and to endure longer as champions. Ed Corney, the splendid body on the cover of *Pumping Iron* and on all the movie posters, is in his mid-forties, and he's still at the top.

As Geng points out, there appears to be no such thing as a generation gap in the world of bodybuilding, since so many ages are represented. And the discipline of working out seems to retard the aging process.

History of Weight-Training
Using weights to increase strength has been around for a long time. Milo of Crotona, an inventive Greek of ancient times, is generally credited with having developed the first "course" in progressive weight-training. His favorite exercise consisted of lifting a calf every day. As the animal grew in size, the man increased in strength. He apparently continued until the calf became a full-grown bull — no light feat. That this training worked is proved by the fact that he won many championships in the Olympics over a period of forty years.

In his book *Weight Training for Athletes*, Bob Hoffman describes how Roman soldiers went through a sort of basic training that involved weights.[16] This included running, jumping, and swimming "while carrying stones and bars of metal." They exercised their arms with "sticks laden at either end with stones"; in effect, these contraptions were the first dumbbells.

Hoffman says that the first person who did weight-training is assumed to have lived "in a land at the eastern end of the Mediterranean Sea. Historians and archeologists have found evidence that the ancient Egyptians, Persians, Medes, and Babylonians all held stones and leaded objects in their hands while practicing for jumping and running." It's recorded that athletes prepared with weights for the first Olympic Games, in 776 B.C.

Much later, Elizabethan archers caught on to weight-training as a way to improve their distance. Hoffman says that the poet John Milton and, even earlier, author Sir Thomas Elyot advised all Englishmen to train with weights. European armies trained that way for centuries.

So much for ancient weightlifting. As for the beginnings of modern practice, Jim Murray and Peter Karpovich outline its history in their book *Weight Training in Athletics*. During the 19th Century "untold numbers of professional strongmen lifted their barbells and performed spectacular stunts with carnivals and on vaudeville stages. Most of them got their starts in amateur clubs, often in the back rooms of taverns where vigorous young men met to wrestle, box, and lift weights."[17] Sort of like modern men's clubs.

The problem was one of technology: the weights were extremely cumbersome. "Iron globes were cast with iron or steel connecting bars, and other weights were cast as single globes or blocks with projecting handles."[18] Ironically, since the weights were fixed, and therefore heavy from the start (as opposed to modern, adjustable weights), before anyone could begin to lift weights, he already had to be pretty damn strong! That's how Murray and Karpovich explain why it was only relatively recently that "weights came into use as a strengthener of the person below par physically."

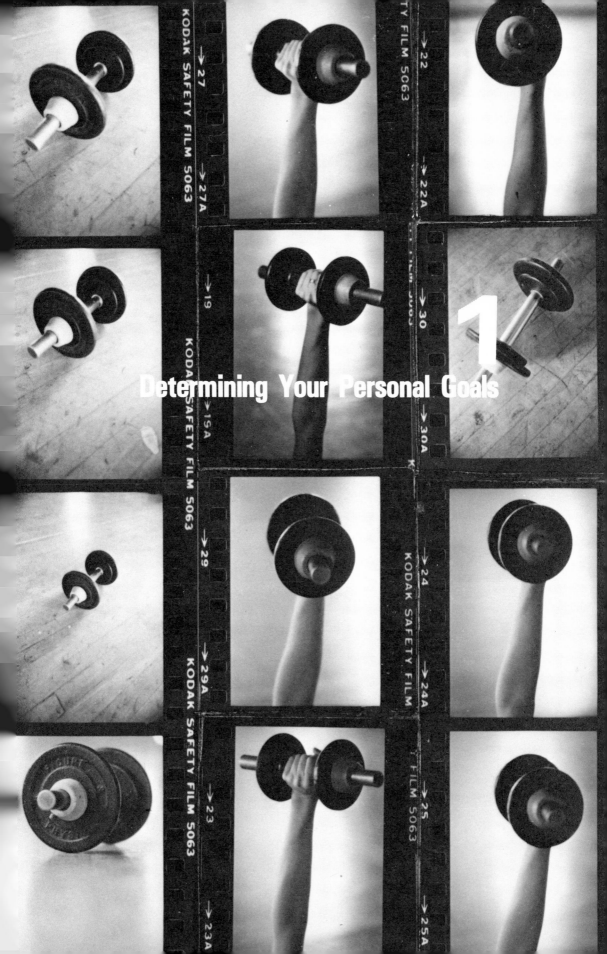

1
Determining Your Personal Goals

What's in It for You?

The question to ask yourself at the start is: what do I want out of this? A few people weight-train for the express purpose of competing in those sports that involve the lifting of weights or to compete in bodybuilding contests. A lot more do it to improve their performance in a specific sport — like tennis or running — or to make them more fit to carry out activities related to work or domestic life (like carrying an infant). Many others do it to lose or gain weight, and to improve their appearance. Some do it to become stronger and more self-confident and to improve their status in a shakey physical world.

In responding to a survey by Bill Reynolds, a majority of 200 bodybuilders revealed that they started the sport as adolescents — after seeing an ad of the Charles Atlas type or reading the back of a cereal box that promoted "he-men." They figured they wanted to be big and strong and decided they'd better work at it, since they were at an age when they were feeling insecure about how their bodies would develop. So there is naturally both an offensive and a defensive rationale in their taking up body-building. No boy wants to be the skinny, gutless guy who gets sand kicked in his face at the beach. Everyone wants to be the admired lifeguard.

Women tend to have a common goal of wanting to look better, by toning their bodies and trimming fat. And both female and male athletes put weight-training on their agenda to improve strength, dexterity, and to prevent or rehabilitate injuries.

It's up to you to decide what you want to accomplish. Once you decide, give yourself enough time to reach that goal. If you have a definite goal, e.g., you want to trim your waist, it's best to set a series of gradual goals. Rather than swearing you're going to lose six inches in the next year, tell yourself you're going to lose a half inch in the next month. This is a perfectly reasonable goal, provided you train regularly and eat sensibly. Then measure yourself in a month's time to see if you've accomplished this goal. Solid changes take time, so don't measure yourself every day.

Side Benefits

When you become stronger, a lot of other good things happen to you. It isn't just a matter of being able to lift more weight or to exert more force. As Bob Hoffman says, "It also means a more efficient distribution and use of the elements of energy and repair."[1] That's how weight-training makes you more fit and able to withstand stress and avert possible injuries. Being in better shape means your body is more able to cope with problems that may confront it.

Different Strokes for Different Folks

One thing to keep in mind, especially if you're planning to train with someone else, is that not everyone progresses at the same rate. We've already discussed the different potentials of men and women. Even two people of the same sex, age, body weight, and height, following identical training programs, may still experience different rates of progress. It's not completely understood why, but it does appear that some people make easier gains than others. It's like how different people have different metabolic rates for reasons beyond our ken.

The exercises in this book take into account different capabilities by suggesting pound-ages in terms of your sex and body weight. Don't worry: you won't be asked to do as much as a person twice your size. And ranges of repetitions (how many times you perform each exercise) are given, so you can personalize the exercises even further.

Tightening Up Doesn't Mean Becoming Uptight

An intriguing aspect of weight-training is how close it gets to welding together body and soul. At its best, any activity in life should do that, I suppose. But I found the special charm of the book *Pumping Iron* to be the authors' ability to capture the mystical aspects of such a vigorously physical and misunderstood activity. As he they quote Ed Corney: "Most people think that bodybuilders are strictly after their body in appearance only. I find . . . that's only half of it. The other half is it comes on rather strong in developing yourself mentally as well. A broad outlook on life — the trials and tribulations, ups and downs, you know. You're able to take things as they come and go."[2]

The thing that boggles the mind (or should I say body?) is how weight-training, of all the sports or exercises I can think of, gets directly to the body. There's no middle ground and no messenger service. You can work actively and directly on sculpting your body — building this muscle, refining that one, slimming one body part or building up another.

When practiced with respect, seriousness, and a balanced perspective, weight-training can become a high art form. It is like ballet, gymnastics, tennis, skiing, skating, or any other physical activity that segues into art when executed with style, grace, and excellence.

Many professionals with high-pressure jobs that exhaust their minds are finding weight-training to be the perfect outlet for expressing the physical self. It grinds out worries while building in strength. Doing the exercises provides a psychological lift, and there comes an incredible sense of power in knowing that you've got control over your body, that you can make it grow or diminish and look the way you want. Your attitude about your body changes: it's no longer just this thing you live in that you tend, like a house with a leaky roof or a broken window, only when something goes wrong.

So if you've ever had sand kicked in your face, if you're often afraid that you wouldn't be able to defend yourself against a mugger, if you feel your body is deteriorating with age, if you have to struggle just to open the catsup bottle, if you wheeze and ache from lugging groceries upstairs, if you want to improve your tennis backhand, if you want to run a faster mile, if you want to put more spring into your legs for basketball or volleyball, weight-training can do wonders for you. It will very likely raise your spirits, besides, and help you look at your entire life style in a more healthful light. Don't be surprised if you also start improving your nutrition, your sleeping habits, and your work schedule.

The Inner Game of Weight-Training

Robert Abraham Zuver is the forty-seven-year-old owner of Zuver's Gym Equipment, Factory and Showroom in Southern California. He is a bodybuilder, artist, and an ordained United Fundamentalist minister. A potpourri of sensibilities, he likes to think of himself as an "athletic chaplain." As macho as a man can get on the one hand (he can lift 500 pounds), Zuver is still aware of the yin-yang, male-female forces that allow a man to be strong, yet sensitive. He says, "Being manly and being strong certainly doesn't mean that you've got to be brutey and . . . heavy in your speech towards everything and in your mannerisms."[3]

Although his business is merchandising physical fitness, Zuver insists that fitness alone, as a commodity or as a goal, has no innate value. "Fitness can only be spelled out in one way, and that's mental, physical, and spiritual balance. If you can't teach the whole thing, you can't teach it at all. The reason you can't teach it at all is because you can't separate them . . . . We're not all mental, we're not all spiritual, we're not all physical." Amen.

On Losing Weight

It is quite possible to lose weight while weight-training, but you must modify your diet. This book does not recommend any particular diet, but one key to dieting is to reduce the amount of food you eat. This may mean eating less of everything, cutting out certain kinds of foods, or eating fewer meals. A high-protein diet, low in fat and carbohydrates, is often recommended by nutritionists.

If you are serious about losing weight and would like weight-training to help you reach your goal, you should faithfully adhere to a three-day-a-week program, concentrate on exercises that work the bigger muscle groups (this burns up more calories), and — *this is very important* — regularly do an aerobic exercise, e.g., run, swim, or cycle. Doing a hundred sit-ups will not accomplish what an aerobic will, and exercising specific areas will do less for losing weight than running. Running doesn't work directly on a pudgy stomach, but in the long run (pun intended) including it in your overall exercise program will get you better long-term, all-around results.

What knocks off fat is exercise that burns up a lot of calories. In weight-training that means exercises for the leg and back will be more beneficial (they work bigger muscle groups) than those for the arms and stomach. One way to find out which ones use the most calories is to go through a program and see which exercises make you work the hardest (and probably feel the worst). You'll likely find they include exercises like squats, leg presses, bentover rows, and power cleans.

The concept of "foot-pounds" may be helpful here. There's a direct relationship between calories expended and foot-pounds used. For example, if you move a 50-lb. weight two feet, that's 100 foot-pounds per repetition. When you do light weights in high repetitions, you can accumulate more foot-pounds than if you use a very heavy weight a few times. (In other words, you can do 50 lbs. ten times — that's 500 foot-pounds — but you can probably do 100 lbs. only three or four times, which means 300-400 foot-pounds.) You can keep track of your total tonnage as a way of measuring your progress.

When you lose weight, you lose it everywhere. You can't direct your body to get rid of the fat in just your thighs and your cheeks. Of course, you should exercise specific problem areas to help tone them up while you're in the process of losing weight. The chances are that if you have an especially fatty area, e.g., thighs, the weight loss there will be more dramatic, and you should firm it up through exercise.

For a full explanation of the weight loss program, please see Chapter 5.

On Gaining Weight

The same basic principles that apply to losing weight apply to gaining weight. You will have to adjust your diet; in the case of gaining weight, this means taking in more food. Bill Reynolds says a good rule to follow is to never allow yourself to get hungry; feel free to snack on healthy things between meals. (Please note gaining weight doesn't mean junking it up with potato chips, candy bars, and beer.)

If you want to gain weight and muscle mass, do a few basic exercises with very heavy weights, low repetitions, and a high number of sets. And avoid doing more than one abdominal exercise per workout. The whole idea of increasing weights is to increase muscle size, which will result in weight gain.

See the program for gaining weight in Chapter 5.

Miscellaneous Goals and Misconceptions

Women often express an interest in developing their breasts. Actually, those exercise devices that are advertised to put ten inches on your bust in five hours are basically resistance training devices. But the truth is: no, you can't get bigger breasts. What you *can* do is develop your chest, so that your breasts are better supported and defined. And a woman who fears she is overdeveloped will benefit by strengthening her chest wall and shoulders for better support of heavy breasts. Your bra size might actually increase from weight-training, but this will be due to the development of your back muscles.

As for men who wish to develop their . . . private parts. Sorry, but that's not a muscle.

Mirror, Mirror on the Wall . . .

Bodybuilders, because they're always looking at themselves in mirrors, are often accused of being narcissistic. But this is essential in their training. Their goal is to sculpt themselves, and not to watch what they're doing to themselves would be like any sculptor working blindfolded. It's an excellent idea to watch yourself in a mirror while you do the exercises — just like dancers watch themselves as they rehearse — to be sure you're using proper form, and to watch your body go through some intriguing changes.

If you want to keep track of your progress, buy a little notebook and record your workouts (see the sample format given in Chapter 6) or measure yourself at the beginning and end of each new program. But the best way to tell how you're doing is to size yourself up in a mirror periodically. You can also snap Polaroids of yourself . . . before and after.

Also, notice how much easier it is to lift things around the house. And see how your performance in sports improves. Have your tennis strokes become more powerful? Are you hitting more consistent base-line drives? Aren't you making those strikes in bowling with a little more confidence and power? When you hike, don't your legs seem to hold up longer? Listen for compliments from other people about how you look, how you've changed. And be alert to the fact that you're probably more energetic and really awake, when awake, and soundly asleep when asleep.

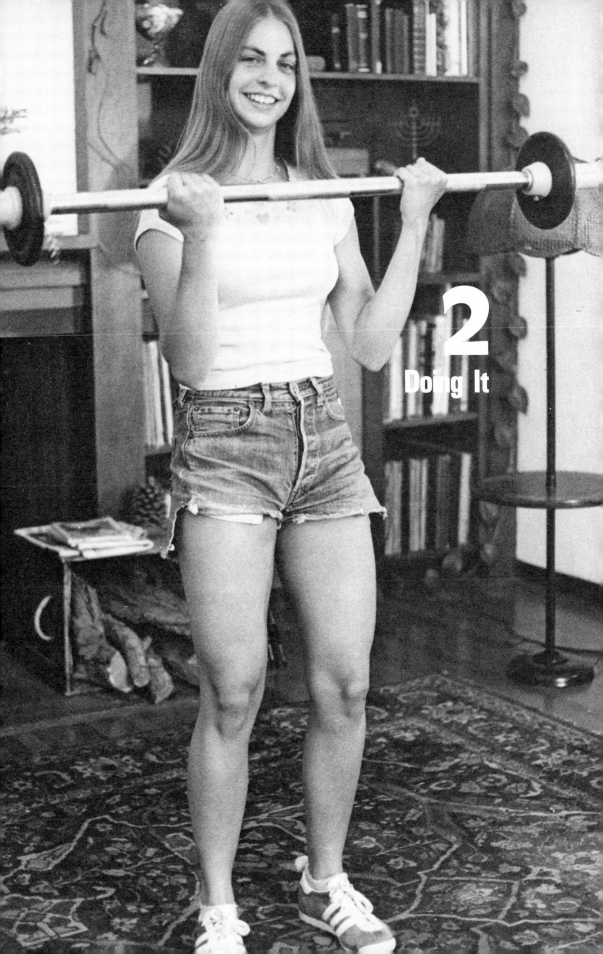

2
Doing It

Pumping Iron?

When we speak of the "pump" in weight-training, we're not referring to a device you find at a gas station, a kind of shoe, or a contraption used to get water out of the earth.

In weight-training terms, the pump is the reaction of your body to the vigorous exercise of a particular muscle.

Philip Rasch explains that "muscles may be regarded as machines which store chemical energy and convert it to mechanical work in response to impulses conducted by the nervous system. There are approximately 434 muscles, making up 40-50 percent of the body weight, but only about 75 pairs are involved in the general movements of the body." He describes how one becomes stronger and possibly bigger by weight-training:

> When a muscle is exercised, the material enclosing the cell becomes thickened and toughened and the amount of connective tissue increases. There is also an increase in certain chemical constituents of the cell, the blood flow, and the blood pressure. The capillaries (tiny blood vessels) open and dilate, and fluid is attracted from the blood into the tissue spaces. All this may increase the weight of the muscle by as much as 20 percent.[1]

When you work a muscle, energy is formed by an interaction of oxygen, glycogen, and other muscle fuels. This creates energy and waste products (carbon dioxide and fatigue toxins). When you exercise, your muscles get larger because of the increased flow of blood that rushes in to replenish fuel and oxygen and to remove waste products. This temperary increase, or swelling, is what we mean by "the pump." After a while, things simmer down: these processes are completed so your blood flow returns to normal. Thus, your muscle doesn't actually grow while you're exercising, although it appears to. Real muscle growth actually takes place between your workout sessions, when you're resting.

After you're through exercising, the muscle will reduce in size, but for a while it will tend to stay bigger than it was before you exercised. So if you continue to work out regularly, and especially if you increase the resistance (the number of pounds you lift), your muscles will get bigger or stay the same, depending on what you want — increased strength or maintenance of fitness.

An increase in strength is based on the "overload" principle: this means you have to keep increasing the weights in order to develop your muscles. Your body will adapt itself to increased stress, and unless you up the ante on your muscles, they will not become stronger. That's not to say you won't maintain your current shape or that it's bad for you not to increase. But you won't progress unless you continue to overload your muscles and force them to work a little harder. Bill Reynolds says that as soon as an exercise becomes too comfortable, it's time to move on . . . to increase the number of times you do it or the poundage you're using.

As your exercised muscles grow stronger, they're more able to accommodate the demands you place on them. They respond to being pushed. So if it's greater strength you're after — and even just plain fitness — it's the last two or three repetitions of an exercise that count the most. Just when you're ready to quit, tell yourself that those tough ones are the ones that will get you where you want to go. Psych yourself up. A *little* pain is okay: it means you're really pushing and trying.

How to Get Started

The first thing you have to decide is·where you want to train. You have several options. You can do it at home. You can join a commercial spa, health club, or gym. You can become a member of the local YMCA or YWCA. You may arrange to use a high school or college weight room.

There are advantages and disadvantages to all these options. Commercial spas and clubs, which tend to be expensive, are geared somewhat to the comfort and ease of more affluent customers, but the expensive dues you pay help to buy some very nice equipment and probably lots of room in which to work out. The environment is likely to be pleasant, with plenty of mirrors and other extras to make the experience more enjoyable. Y's and commercial gyms generally have good equipment, and their charges for membership are reasonable. But you have to adapt to their limited hours, their limited space, and their location (Y's are not known for being in the best neighborhood in town). Depending on the number of members, you may have to wait your turn to use certain equipment. School weight rooms are excellent places to train, depending on the school's budget. Because of the importance of weight-training in sports, they generally have good equipment and good instructors. And there are many people around who know what they're doing, so you won't lack sources of information. The problem, of course, is that you have to be a student or faculty member (or maybe a patronizing alumnus) to qualify to use these facilities.

So that leaves home. This book assumes that for most people it's most convenient to work out at home at least when they're starting out.

Training at home provides the advantages of privacy and convenience. You can do it at your leisure, and you never have to worry about competing for use of equipment. You will have to acquire the necessary equipment, of course, and you'll need a little bit of space in which to work out. These shouldn't be much of a problem. The expense is rather modest, and the necessary space can be found in the living room, bedroom, family room, garage — or any odd corner of the house. You won't be able to buy the amount of equipment that a gym or spa would offer, but you won't have to pay their membership fees either. The fact is you can get along very well at home for the first year of your training, using a minimum of basic equipment, on a relatively small investment. If you decide to join a gym or some other facility later, your equipment at home will still be useful when you work on a more advanced schedule or on those days when you can't get to the gym.

Basic Equipment

The basic equipment needed for weight-training includes: a set of adjustable barbells, a set of adjustable dumbbells, a bench (you can improvise one), and possibly iron boots. If you're doing the exercises on a floor that might get scratched by the weights, you should also have handy a mat or old rug.

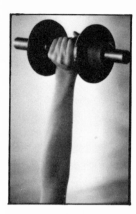 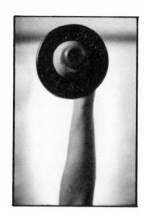 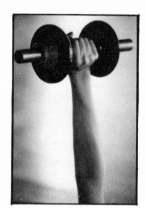

Barbells and dumbbells can be purchased either in an adjustable set or as fixed weights (which means you can't take them apart to accommodate different weights. The bottom line is that you'd have to buy many different sets in order to work with different amounts of weight.)

The barbell is the absolutely basic piece of equipment. If you can't afford anything else, get an adjustable barbell. These come in a variety of lengths and are made of a variety of materials. Length and material determine the weight of a given bar. It is very important to know what it weighs, as this is your basic unit. Don't rely on what you are told when you buy a bar. Weigh it yourself on a bathroom scale. Then there

are the various weight plates that you add. Most adjustable barbells have a sleeve that fits over the bar. This is a hollow metal tube that makes it easier for the bar to revolve when you're changing hand positions. Finally, there are the collars to hold the weight plates in place. You should know the weights of all these components.

Barbell plates are usually heavy iron or semi-steel, and they are made to fit easily on the bar. The more modern ones you see at chic sports stores are colorful and consist of a vinyl covering over concrete or sand. They look pretty and won't scratch your floors, but they're not as durable as metal plates and can be very bulky. Barbell plates come in all weights, from 1¼ lbs. up to 100 lbs.

Dumbbells are constructed of the same materials as barbells. They are much shorter, since you usually use one in each hand. A dumbbell (unloaded) generally weighs 5 lbs.

For beginning and intermediate purposes, you should be able to get by with a 100-125 lb. barbell-dumbbell set. This might run anywhere from $20 to $60, depending on where you buy your equipment. You can purchase weights at stores that specialize in bodybuilding equipment, in sporting goods stores, from mail-order companies, at department stores with athletic departments, or from the want ads. You can try advertising in one of those neighborhood shopper newsletters, where you may be able to get some very good used weights for 10¢ a pound. Don't be put off by rusty metal plates; all you have to do is clean them up and spray paint them. They'll be as good as new.

Among other equipment that can make your workouts more productive and convenient are iron boots, which resemble sandals made of iron. They usually weigh 5 lbs. and can accommodate additional weight plates. If you can't locate a pair, you can do the exercises that call for them with heavy ski boots. Wood blocks also come in handy; you will notice that some of the exercises call for you to elevate your heels. If you don't have any two-by-fours or four-by-fours, a pair of barbell plates or a book of the right thickness will substitute nicely. A small, narrow bench also makes exercising much easier. Its size should depend on your size. You should be able to lie down on it with your head on one hand, your thighs resting comfortably on the bench, your knees bent, and your feet square on the floor. It should generally be about 18" high, 4' long, and 16-20" wide.

Machines

Although this book is designed to be used with free weights (a barbell, dumbbells, and iron boots), you should be aware that there are exercise machines available at spas and gyms. Most institutions feature a variety of machines and pulleys: including isokinetic, calf, leg-press, hack slide, lat, and sliding-press machines. You'll see leg extension/leg curls. There will be various wall, ceiling, and floor pulleys. Incline benches and boards and decline benches and boards can be very helpful, as well as T-bars for rowing, preacher benches, isometric racks, dip bars, and chinning bars.

The most popular kinds of machines are the Universal Gym and the Nautilus. The Universal has been described as a "jungle gym for adults." Diana Nyad goes on to call it "one large mass of steel bars and weighted plates on pulleys that allows an athlete to work different parts of the body on the same machine."

The Nautilus machine is the current rage. It is expensive (you need about twelve to fifteen different devices in order to work all your body parts), but can be found in the spiffier spas and athletic training centers. Nautilus clinics have been opened to cater to the specific needs of athletes. The San Jose Sunbirds, a team in the Women's Professional Softball League, train at a Nautilus center in Cupertino, California, known as SMART (Sports Medicine Athletic Rehabilitation & Training).

The benefits of the Nautilus are actually a matter of debate. Some claim that these machines allow a 25-percent greater range of muscular movement. A definite advantage offered by both the Universal and the Nautilus over free weights is that they're time-saving (you don't have to fiddle around with adjusting weights and moving from station to station). And you don't have to worry about falling barbells or dumbbells.

They are expensive, however (especially the Nautilus), and they take up a lot of room. Free weights are favored by such athletes as Maren Seidler, U.S. shotput champion, who has weight-trained since she was a child. She has developed a very vigorous weight-training program, using both a Nautilus routine and free weights. But, as Diana Nyad puts it, "Seidler vows she will never entirely replace free weights with machines because the coordination required by them duplicates that of the shotput."

Another disadvantage of machines is that *they* control the weights — not you. So, in an athletic context, movements used with free weights more closely approximate realistic circumstances. With a Nautilus, you're always working in a fixed arc when lifting a weight. And from a general standpoint, the greater the variety of angles from which you work a muscle, the better the quality of your development and the greater your improvement. In addition, machines are less versatile than free weights. The Nautilus, for example, might have only two or three exercises for the biceps, while Bill Reynolds claims that with a set of dumbbells he can supply *30* different exercises for the biceps.

Given an ideal situation — barring considerations of expense and assuming you have enough room and time — you probably will want to train with a combination of free weights and machines.

What to Wear
The best clothes to wear for your workouts won't get you on the "Best Dressed" list (although you might have noticed that recent issues of fashion magazines have featured "action" clothes aimed at the fitness market). The important thing is to wear loose, comfortable clothing that will let your body move and sweat. Of course, the weather or the temperature of your training area will affect what you wear. You may prefer to wear as little as possible — that's fine, provided it's warm enough to make you sweat.

Basic gear might consist of a T-shirt, shorts, tennis shoes, and socks. This goes for both men and women, although women might prefer to wear a leotard. Men may also wish to wear a jock strap, and women a bra. (You will notice that some models in our illustrations are not wearing shirts, but that was to exhibit their musculature.)

It's very important (more about this later) to keep warm while exercising, in order to prevent injury and to make you more flexible. So you may want to start out each workout wearing a sweat jacket and/or pants. Exercising affects more than just isolated muscles. Your internal organs become stimulated at the same time — this is why you should be sweating . . . a lot. If you're not, either you're not working hard enough, or the temperature of your training area is too low. In either case, you should correct the situation.

As for wearing shoes, they are a precaution in case you drop a weight (rare, but a possibility). Also, as you advance to heavier poundages, having good arch support becomes important. When working with iron boots, you may find it more comfortable to wear them over shoes.

Warming Up, Warming Down, Keeping Warm

Bill Reynolds likens the human body to an automobile. It requires a warm-up period before it can work at its peak. "A proper warm-up speeds up the pulse rate, makes muscle and connective tissues more pliable and resistant to injury, and actually allows one to lift heavier weights than would be possible without a warm-up."

Lifting weights is far more strenuous than most mundane activities you tackle. So you do have to prepare your body properly. Jumping rope and running in place are excellent warm-up activities. The "clean and press" is usually suggested as the first weight-training exercise in a program. You can also do sit-ups. And there are the stretching exercises that should be done prior to a workout.

You'll know you're properly warmed up if you feel awake, fresh, and ready to go ahead with your workout. You should feel loose and supple. You might even be sweating already. Training without warming up is definitely unwise, as it's dangerous (you're more susceptible to injury when you're cold and brittle). A proper warm-up will also make your muscles more flexible and able to function with less strain.

As you work out, be aware of your body temperature. This is true even when you're resting — don't let yourself cool off in those rest periods. A room temperature of at least 68° F is recommended by the experts.

Warming down is also important — physically and psychologically. It gives your body a chance to gradually wind down and taper off from your workout. Since you would have worked your muscles pretty hard by then, warm-down exercises should be less strenuous than warm-ups.

Stretching

Before you begin your weight-training exercises and even on your days off, you should do about ten minutes of stretching. As Bob Hoffman puts it:

A muscle is similar to a rubber band. Being elastic it can be contorted out of its relaxed shape and then returned to normal. This holds true for ordinary stretching and twisting activities — with one exception: if systematically stretched over a period of time, it will retain an increased ability to stretch. It will become more elastic in the same way that a new rubber band will increase in elasticity with stretching.[2]

If you stretch properly, your body will be more flexible and supple and the exercises will be easier to perform. Also, you'll be able to exercise with better form. And you'll avoid even more the possibility of injury.

Flexibility, of course, plays an important role in sports. Being able to extend yourself just a little bit more, to switch positions rapidly, and to stay loose can be critical in any competition.

The key to good stretching is to complete the motion slowly. Exercise your patience as well. To while away the time while you're stretched out in a particular position, you can read a book, watch TV, listen to the radio, or meditate. Yoga is an excellent complement to weight-training. If you're not a practitioner, turn to the simple stretching exercises described at the end of Chapter 4.

When to Train

You'll find that exercising depresses your appetite (this is terrific if you want to lose weight). So if you don't want it to interfere with your normal meal time, you should work out at least a couple of hours before you plan to eat. You don't want to work out right after you've eaten either, since your blood is busy digesting all that food. Exercising *then* only places unnecessary demands on your body. It's best to wait at least an hour after eating, if not two, before working out.

Everybody has a favorite time to train. You'll discover your own. Franco Columbu suggests training between three and six in the afternoon. This is six to eight hours after most people wake up, and the body is warmed up from activity, yet not wiped out from fatigue.[3]

It's best to experiment, to see how your body responds at different times of the day or night, then establish a regular training time. Your body will begin to gear itself up to a regular workout at that time each day, and it will adjust its natural energy cycles for optimal performance at that time. The end result: a more energetic and productive training session.

If you are using weight-training primarily as a supplement to your regular workout for a specific sport, you should train after you've done your other workout. The idea is to place priorities on your energy: give your best shot to whatever's most important to you. If you have a lot of time to train, then you can weight-train first, but you should do it at least two hours before your other workout to give you a chance to rest up for your next activity.

How Often to Train

What's been found to be most effective (for strange and mysterious reasons, even to physiologists) is three nonconsecutive days of training a week. Most often, this means Monday, Wednesday, and Friday. But there's no reason why it can't be Tuesday, Thursday, and Saturday, or some other combination.

When you're first starting out, you should avoid training two days in a row. You might feel terrific and especially enthusiastic after seeing the first dramatic improvements, but in the long run remember that it's better for the body to have a day in between to rest. Your body needs time to recuperate. Without rest, the muscles can become tired and possibly damaged. On your rest days, you can do an aerobic exercise or play your favorite sport.

If you miss a day, you can work two days in a row to make it up (after you've broken yourself in), especially if what you're after is fitness rather than strength or increased muscle mass. There are still those who maintain that it is during the rest periods that the body actually builds itself, tearing down muscle and rebuilding it into bigger and better chemistry for your body. One bodybuilder, Joe Disco, swears he can hear himself growing during the last three of his twelve hours of sleep — and that it sounds like "cornflakes being poured into a bowl." [4]

It's also important to take a week's layoff every few months. (Most people will naturally do this, as their bodies tell them it's time for a breather.) This gives your body a chance to rest and reconsolidate (perhaps mending minor injuries), but it has an even more important mental effect. It'll give you a chance to miss weight-training and to come back to it with new verve and determination.

How Long to Train

Overtraining can become a problem. By this, I mean that some people rush the process and accelerate their rate of progress to the point of overtaxing their bodies. A weight-training session should last from 45 minutes to an hour, including stretching, warming up, and warming down. If you feel absolutely exhausted at the end of a session, you should probably lighten your exercise load. Feeling used and tired is okay, but those feelings of exhaustion should be accompanied by a sense of exhilaration and accomplishment. You shouldn't be just flat-out fatigued. You should feel up to doing something else afterwards, instead of wanting to sack out.

If you work your body too hard over a period of time, you will exhibit symptoms of overtraining: a lack of enthusiasm when it's time to train, a consistent feeling of dragginess or tiredness, loss of appetite, insomnia, restlessness, and sore muscles all of the time.

If you find yourself with several of these symptoms, you should take a week off to reconsolidate your body and to restructure your program. Examine your attitude about training. Maybe don't be so grim about it: try to approach each workout with a sense of fun and personal achievement. Keep a record of your progress, and congratulate yourself on improvements.

In other words, be more moderate, relaxed, and patient with yourself. Don't try to rebuild yourself in a day.

Warding Off Boredom

It's one thing to raise your consciousness about the benefits of exercise, and quite another to get your body raised and into training every other day. It's like getting on a diet or cutting out smoking. There's a point when you become committed to it, and the unnatural thing would be *not to* train.

But, frankly, weight-training can become boring. Because the workouts are based on repeating the same exercises and because the work is demanding, you may find your attention wandering and your interest fading. There are some preventive measures. Train to music that energizes you, that puts you into the mood. Wear a special T-shirt that inspires you (bodybuilders have collections of these T-shirts). Reorganize your routine *at least* once every ten weeks, preferably every four to six weeks. Train with someone else to keep you company and to inject some competitiveness into your training session. Redefine your goals, and then keep track of your progress. Change the order of the exercises (just to be sure follow the general rules for the order of which body parts to exercise first). Take an occasional week off — this will be a terrific reward (unless you find yourself missing it too much). As I said earlier, this layoff may actually promote better workouts when you resume your training because your body's had a chance to reconsolidate and your mind has been allowed to relax.

Working Through Soreness

Depending on the shape you're in when you first begin to weight-train, you might develop some or a lot of soreness. Pay attention to what your body says. While it's perfectly normal to expect some soreness at first and when you're increasing poundages, don't overdo your training by placing unrealistic stress on your body. The whole point of weight-training is to revitalize you — not to incapacitate you.

When you first begin, or when you resume training after a layoff, break in slowly. Use light weights. And do only one set of each exercise the first time, maybe even the second (despite what your program might say). Be sure to do stretching exercises to increase your flexibility.

Don't be unduly alarmed by a *moderate* amount of soreness. The reason your body responds so achingly is that it isn't accustomed to such hard work and therefore is not efficiently eliminating fatigue toxins from your body. As Bill Reynolds explained to me, "Toxins like lactic acid are not flushed from the muscles, and it's these toxins that cause pain."

If you've ever started any sport, e.g., tennis or skiing, after a period of relative inactivity, you probably can recall experiencing the same kind of muscle soreness. The thing to remember is that this soreness is temporary; it will go away rather quickly — especially if you keep working out. Do not give up just because you feel some aches and pains. If you wait too long between workouts, you'll just have to go through the breaking-in process all over again. What you have to do is to get your body accustomed to being efficient. Fortunately it adapts very quickly by beginning to eliminate the toxins. After a certain amount of training, you will notice less and less soreness.

In the meantime, if you are suffering from soreness and want to alleviate some of the pain, there are some steps you can take. You can get a massage. It may be painful, but you'll get back into training very quickly. Take a hot bath or get into a whirlpppl — this will make you feel better instantly. Sleep on a toasty, heated waterbed. Or, if you're really anxious to get rid of the soreness and get back into the swing of things, do the same workout two days in a row. This will hurt, since you're still sore, but it will force your body to act more efficiently immediately — and get rid of those toxins that are causing the pain.

As Franco Columbu writes in *Winning Bodybuilding,* pay attention to which of your muscles become sore and which ones actually cause pain. "The difference is quite simple; while this sounds strange to say, muscle soreness is not unpleasant at all. You get accustomed to it quickly during training, and learn to look for it as a sign that your training is really working. Pain, on the other hand, is enjoyed only by a weird few, and is a legitimate and certain signal that something is wrong."[5]

If you suspect that you have injured yourself — if you suffer from hard-core pain rather than mere soreness — you should see a doctor or someone else who can treat your problem. There's no sense in playing the martyr or in being bashful about reporting your pain.

Proper Form — Go with a Flow

Doing the exercises a million times and with a thousand tons won't do you a bloody bit of good unless you do them properly. This is why it's a good idea when you're starting out to watch yourself in a mirror, or have someone (preferably a person who knows how to weight-train) observe you to make sure you get started off on the right foot.

You should start each exercise slowly and deliberately. The tempo — how fast you do the exercise — can be stepped up as you reach the end of your set. This means that the final three or four repetitions can be done with a little more speed. Just don't get sloppy about your form.

Basic Definitions

So that you can understand the program prescriptions and exercises, here is a brief glossary of common terms used:

Repetition: Each time you perform an exercise. The number of repetitions in a set can range anywhere from 5 to 100.

Set: A group of repetitions of an exercise. You will usually perform from one to five sets of an exercise.

Overgrip: While standing erect holding a barbell across your thighs, your palms are facing your legs.

Undergrip: In the same position as above, your palms are facing away from your legs.

Mixed Grip: One hand in an overgrip, the other in an undergrip.

Clean: To pull the weight from the floor to your chest in one movement.

Power Clean: To pull the weight from the floor to your chest, then jump under it and pull it all the way up to arms' length.

Snatch: To pull the weight from the floor to arms' length overhead in one motion, while splitting or squatting under it.

Power Snatch: To pull the weight from the floor to arms' length overhead in one motion, without splitting or squatting under it.

Press: To push the weight away from your body at arms' length — standing, lying down, or seated.

Doing the exercises slowly and with a steady rhythm is critical. Sudden, jerky movements mean you're probably working the wrong muscles. And there's also the chance you'll injure yourself this way. Evelyn Hsu theorizes that her beginning students exhibit painful expressions because of the Puritan ethic. They feel it should hurt while they're exercising, so they fling themselves about.

Concentrate on moving the weight along the full range of motion described in the exercise recipe. Don't cut any movements short. Don't ever end an exercise or work-out abruptly.

Proper form will develop the greatest strength, so look at it as a matter of pure economy to be graceful and methodical. You'll get more out of the time you're invest-ing in weight-training if you do ti right. Philip Rasch maintains that "mechanical efficiency is greatest at about one-fifth of the maximal speed. The movements should be made slowly and steadily, with the final position held firmly for a few seconds."[6]

Even if you're exercising quickly (which is perfectly all right, as long as you use a con-sistent tempo), the movements should be deliberate and steady. Your rests between sets should be in rhythm with your exercise motions; they should fit right into the tempo of your training session.

A good habit to develop right at the beginning is concentration. As you reach more advanced levels of weight-training, you'll find — as bodybuilders do — that it's con-centration that separates the sheep from the goats.

As Charles Gaines observes from his pilgrimage into the bodybuilding world: "Con-centration . . . means thinking a muscle through what it is doing — forcing it with your mind, and with your eyes if you can stare at it, to work fully . . . . All the best body-builders can block out an air war with their concentration."[7]

When working out, focus your attention on the muscle(s) being worked so that you apply stress to the correct area of your body. This can also help to prevent bad form and possible injury. When doing a barbell curl, for example, you should focus on work-ing your biceps, not your legs or back.

All weight-training instructors stress that proper form is every bit as important — if not more so — than the amount of weight you can lift. Slow and steady is infinitely pre-ferable to fast and and jerky. There's no race to win. "Pumping iron" **does not** mean to use a pumping motion. There is a growing number of weight-training experts who believe that in terms of developing strength, *lowering* the weight is every bit as impor-tant as lifting it. Some go so far as to say that lowering is a superior movement for muscular development. At any rate, pay close attention to your recovery (how you return the weight after you've lifted it). It isn't just a matter of getting the weight haphazardly back to where it started, in fact, it's an essential part of the exercise. And slow and steady should be the rule there as well.

There are some bad habits to avoid forming. Don't use the wrong body part when doing an exercise designed for a specific muscle group. Proper concentration will help you work the right muscles. You should also avoid becoming slipshod about maintain-ing your schedule. A regular three-day-a-week schedule is the recommended dosage.

Don't skip workouts unless you absolutely must. And if you do miss any, try to make them up on another day.

Practicing proper form in weight-training can have nice applications to your everyday life, whether you are required to lift such heavy things as infants, bags of groceries, suitcases, crates, portable appliances, work tools, etc. What you learn from weight-training applies to all these other activities: when you lift any heavy object, you should have your feet on the same line, hips lowered, head up, and back straight. Jim Murray and Peter Karpovich maintain that this is the position that places the least amount of strain on your back or abdomen by utilizing the largest and strongest muscles of your body — which happen to be located in your legs and back.[8]

How Much Weight Should You Lift?

Please keep in mind that different individuals vary greatly (depending on their own weight) in terms of how much weight they can handle. respect your limits, especially when you're beginning. Remember that you should determine how much weight to lift for each exercise as *a percentage of your own body weight* — so be sure of what you weigh before loading on the weight plates. And don't be afraid to use a little less if you feel too much stress. Jack Dellinger, former Mr. America and Mr. Universe, advises, "You must use a weight that is light enough so that it will not cause any strain and yet heavy enough so that when the allotted number of . . . repetitions are done you will feel a pumping and swollen feeling in the muscle. Don't confuse strain by the pumping of blood into the muscle tissue. This is quite natural and when you experience this swollen feeling you will know you are exercising correctly."[9]

When you first get this feeling, rejoice — for this is the mythical "pump," about which bodybuilders croon. In the inimitable Arnold Schwarzenegger's words: "A bodybuilder knows that when he pumps up his muscles it means growth . . . he knows when he pumps up well, that is progress. And that satisfies him because he feels that progress in his body. Therefore the pump feels good. It's actually the best feeling a bodybuilder can have. It's a difficult thing to explain. Like sometimes we joke around and we get a good pump and we say you have to admit that a good pump is better than coming."

How to Progress

Since weight-training is based on progressive resistance, increasing the amount of weight you lift is critical to the success of your particular program. How you do it is simple: each time you reach the top suggested number of repetitions (e.g., fifteen) and it becomes comfortable, add some weight and drop the number of repetitions to the lowest suggested number in your next workout.

There are different rules to use for how much weight to add. It depends on whether you're a man or a woman, and whether the exercises involve your upper body (arms, chest) or your legs and back. If the exercise works the upper body, men should be able to increase the poundages by 5 to 10 lbs., while the more powerful legs and back should be able to withstand an increase of 10 to 15 lbs. Women can gauge their increases approximately by using half of the suggested poundages for men.

Adding weights is one way to increase your resistance. Another way is to increase the number of repetitions (which is especially good if you're trying to lose weight). The other possibility is to decrease the length of time you rest between sets.

A combination of all these things is ideal.

Occasionally you will reach plateaus, or "sticking points." You seem to find yourself at a dead end; you feel as if you just can't increase your resistance. One way around this problem is to change the exercise to an equivalent one, e.g., substitute dumbbell presses for barbell presses. The idea is to jolt yourself out of the rut.

Most people will have enough scattered layoffs so they won't increase their resistance beyond what they can manage after around nine months of training. This is fine: it's perfectly okay to ebb and flow, provided you come back to the training. If you don't have too many layoffs, you'll grow gradually stronger *ad infinitum*, assuming you continue an active three-day-a-week training program. If you reach a point where you're very pleased with yourself, you can reduce the number of workouts to two, simply to maintain where you are.

The funny thing is that most people get hooked — and even when they've reached one goal, they want to keep going, improving, getting stronger, and feeling better.

Breathing
There are different schools of thought on how you should breathe while weight-training. The only thing everyone agrees on is that you should breathe. Don't laugh. A common mistake among beginners is to hold their breath while lifting.

Inhaling lets oxygen into your lungs, where it mixes with your blood and then travels to all the cells of your body. This is what gives you energy so that you can weight-train. Exhaling rids you of carbon dioxide and other wastes filtered from the blood stream. As Bill Reynolds succinctly sums it up, there are three basic approaches to breathing:

1. There are those who say you should inhale on the exertion phase of each movement, and exhale on the recovery.

2. There are those who reverse this logic, saying you should inhale on the recovery, and exhale on the exertion.

3. Then there are those (like Reynolds) who maintain, "It doesn't matter. As long as you are taking in the amount of air required, you're doing fine."

You're probably pretty safe going with your natural inclination.

Safety
For the purposes of safety, you should always use collars with your barbell and dumbbells to prevent the weight plates from slipping off. If you exercise with iron boots, be sure the straps are secure.

Once you begin lifting heavier weights, you might also want to wear a weight-lifting belt (it gives abdominal and lower-back stability). And you should use a spotter while doing heavy bench presses and squats. (A spotter can help you out if you get into a crunch and are unable to remove a weight that you are lifting.)

And to avoid injury or strain, you should always do a proper warmup, warm down, and plenty of stretching; wear proper clothing; and work out in a comfortable temperature. You should also avoid placing too much stress on any one body part. Use common sense and intelligence, and follow the guidelines in Chapter 5 when designing your own programs.

3

The Exercises

LIST OF EXERCISES
(Alphabetical Order)

—Barbell Calf Raise (#15)
—Barbell Curls (#35)
—Barbell French Press (#38)
—Bench Press (#27)
—Bench Squat (#4)
—Bent Arm Pullover (#21)
—Bentover Lateral (#34)
—Bentover Rowing (#23)
—Bentover Twisting (#49)
—Calf Raise:
  Barbell (#15)
  Dumbbell (#14)
—Clean & Press (#1)
—Concentration Curls (#37)
—Deadlift (#24)
—Dumbbell Calf Raise (#14)
—Dumbbell Curls (#36)
—Dumbbell French Press (#39)
—Dumbbell Kickback (#40)
—French Press:
  Barbell (#38)
  Dumbbell (#39)
—Front Lateral Raise (#32)
—Front Leg Raise (#7)
—Front Squat (#3)
—Good Morning (#26)
—Jumping Squat (#5)
—Knee-Up (#46)
—Leg Curl (#10)
—Leg Extension (#6)
—Leg Raise (#45)
—Leg Spread (#9)
—Lunge (#11)
—Lying Bent Arm Lateral (#29)

—Lying Straight Arm Lateral (#28)
—Military Press (#30)
—Power Clean (#17)
—Power Snatch (#18)
—Press behind Neck (#31)
—Reverse Curl (#41)
—Reverse Wrist Curl (#43)
—Seated Calf Exercise (#13)
—Self Hand Pressure (#20)
—Shoulder Shrug (#20)
—Sidebend (#47)
—Side Lateral Raise (#33)
—Side Leg Raise (#8)
—Sit-up (#44)
—Squat (#2)
—Step-Up (#12)
—Stiff-Leg Deadlift (#25)
—Straddle Hop (#16)
—Straight Arm Pullover (#22)
—Twisting (#48)
—Upright Rowing (#19)
—Wrestler's Bridge (#50)
—Wrist Curl (#42)

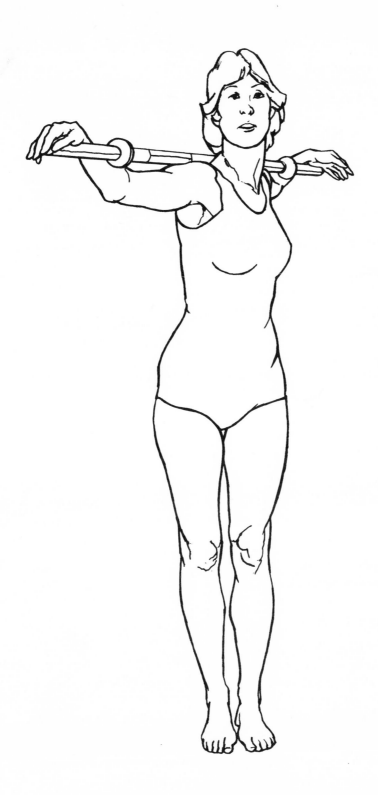

The Exercises

What follows here is an exercise pool, consisting of the exercises that make up the programs presented in the next chapter. You should select a program, then locate the recipe for each exercise in the alphabetical table of exercises (page 34). The exercises are grouped according to which muscle groups they work.

We have divided the body into these general parts: legs, back, chest, shoulders, upper arms, forearms, abdomen, waist, and neck. Of course, many exercises affect more than one of these body parts, but we have listed the exercises according to which body part they affect most. This is to make it easier for you to design your own programs: all you have to do is decide which body parts you want to improve and assemble a balanced group of exercises. (Be sure to read the introduction to Chapter 5 before concocting your own program recipe).

As you will see, each weight-training exercise has been carefully illustrated. Observe the drawings carefully, and make sure you practice proper form from the start. Pay attention to details (such as where your hands and feet start and end up), and be aware of any cautionary notes.

Dumbbells vs. Barbell?
Each exercise lists necessary and optional equipment. Often you can make a choice between using a barbell or dumbbells for a particular exercise. You should try to balance your program with dumbbell exercises because they offer some distinct advantages over a barbell. For instance, when you use a barbell and have a weaker side (most people do), your stronger side automatically assumes more of the load. But if you use dumbbells, this isn't possible. You can't cheat. Each side must share the burden equally. So using dumbbells is a good way to balance your strength and to increase the strength of your weaker side.

Another consideration is that you might actually work the muscles harder with dumbbells. Philip Rasch contends in *Weight Training* that dumbbells often create more stress on the muscles. An example of this is the press, where "the even distribution of the weight on the barbell tends to inhibit any tendency for the bar to move sideways, whereas dumbbells require a powerful contraction of the shoulder muscles to keep them from dropping to the sides. Few individuals can press as much with two dumbbells as they can with one barbell."

Negative Movement & Recovery
Many studies have found that negative movement (eccentric contraction), or how you lower the weight, has as much potential for developing strength as how you lift the weight. Be sure to return the weight slowly, and you will get twice as much out of your workouts. By doing this you also decrease your chances of getting hurt. The upright rowing exercise is a prime example of where you'd be losing half the benefit of an exercise (and subjecting yourself to possible injury) by sloppily dropping the weight back to starting position (rather than resisting it slowly all the way back down).

As for how to return a weight to the starting position so that you can complete the necessary number of repetitions, simply reverse the motions you used to get there.

Foot Stance

In many of the exercise descriptions, you are told to assume a comfortable foot stance. You may want to take into consideration the fact that a narrow foot stance places more stress on your thighs, while a wider one has more effect on your buttocks. So choose your stance accordingly.

Grip Width

Most of the exercises prescribe a certain width of grip. In general, a medium or narrow grip is better than a very wide one. This is because wide grips result in a shorter range of motion. You can see this clearly by standing in front of a mirror and comparing what wide and medium grips allow you to do. It should be obvious that the barbell travels a longer distance with the narrower grip.

Leg Exercises

The legs can be divided into four muscle groups: the *quadriceps* (front of the thigh), the *biceps femoris*, commonly known as the hamstrings (back of the thigh), the hip musculature, and the calves.

Leg exercises include:
1. Clean & Press (total body exercise and ideal warm-up)
2. Squat
3. Front Squat
4. Bench Squat
5. Jumping Squat
6. Leg Extension
7. Front Leg Raise
8. Side Leg Raise
9. Leg Spread
10. Leg Curl
11. Lunge
12. Step-up
13. Seated Calf Exercise
14. Dumbbell Calf Raise
15. Barbell Calf Raise
16. Straddle Hop

Exercise #1: CLEAN & PRESS

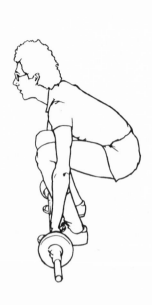 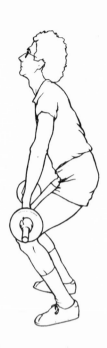 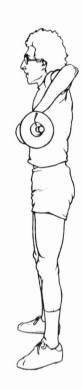

Equipment: Nearly every body part and muscle group, including the thighs, lower back, upper back, biceps, triceps, and upper chest. Calves, abdomen, and grip muscles are used as stabilizers.

General Notes: This is a most effective warm-up exercise, as it combines the clean and the military press. If you were able to do only one weight-training exercise, this would be the one to do. The clean & press should be done with a light weight, as it should be used to stimulate your body for the workout to come where you'll be using heavier weights.

How to Do: A. With the weight on the floor and the bar almost touching your shins, take hold of the barbell with a slightly wider-than-shoulder-width over-grip. Pull it back towards your center of gravity. Be sure to keep your head up and your back straight (do not bow your back). Also, your hips should be kept low and your arms completely extended.

B. Begin to straighten your legs, keeping your back at approximately the same angle. Your arms should still be locked until after the bar passes your knees. The barbell is actually being lifted by your legs.

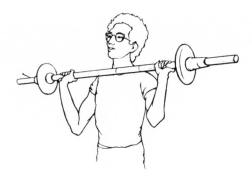

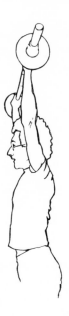

C. As soon as your legs and back are straight, your arms should follow through by pulling up the weight. Your elbows should be pointed up and out to the sides.

D. Whip your elbows forward to cradle the bar at the base of your neck.

E. Keeping your torso erect, push the weight (your palms should be pointed up towards the ceiling) over your head to the full extent of your arms.

Without pausing, return the weight to your chest, then to a position below your knees, and use this as your starting position for each repetition. In other words, you shouldn't set the weight down on the floor until you complete a set.

Cautionary Note: This is a complex exercise, demanding some rather precise movements. To make sure you're doing it properly from the very beginning, get your form checked out by an experienced weight-trainer. And until you're absolutely sure you've got it correctly, watch yourself perform this one in a mirror.

Exercise #2: SQUAT

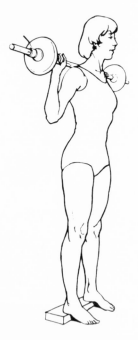

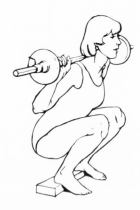

Equipment: Barbell (optional: 2" x 4" board and a weight rack)

Muscles Worked: Lower body muscles in general, including thighs and hips.

General Notes: The squat is basically a knee-bend done with a weight.

When you're first starting out, you'll be able to lift the amount of weight that you can accommodate on your back without assistance. But, as you build strength, You'll soon require another person (a spotter) to help you place the barbell on your shoulders. Or, an alternative at that point is to obtain a weight rack.

You can increase your comfort and maintain your balance better by placing your heels on a 2" x 4" board.

When you graduate to heavier weights, you should pad the bar. A towel will do the job nicely.

How to Do: A. Place a barbell on your shoulders behind your head, and hold it there with a wide overgrip. Stand erect, being sure to keep your back straight and your chest high. Your legs should be comfortably apart, with your toes slightly turned out. To make sure your head and torso stay upright, fix your eyes on a spot on the opposite wall (above eye level) while you're performing this exercise.

B. Tighten your back and leg muscles and lower yourself into a full squat — getting down as low as possible without losing your balance.

Return to the starting position, and repeat.

Cautionary Notes: Somewhere back in the myth-ridden Fifties, squats developed a bad reputation and were blamed for ruining athletes' knees. This notion has since been abandoned by knowledgeable coaches. According to Bill Reynolds, the

Exercise #3: FRONT SQUAT

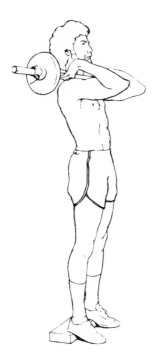

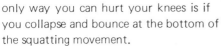

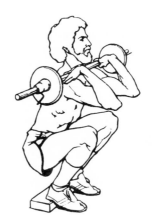

only way you can hurt your knees is if you collapse and bounce at the bottom of the squatting movement.

Equipment: Barbell (optional: 2" x 4" board)

Muscles Worked: Particularly good for thigh muscles just above the knees.

General Notes: This requires the same knee-bend motion as the squat, except that you hold the barbell across your upper chest. The effect of holding the bar in front, rather than behind you, is to give the extensor muscles close to the knees more of the job of keeping your trunk erect. Because it puts a slightly different stress on your legs, you'll probably be able to do a little less (maybe 10-20!) than the regular squat.

How to Do: A. Hold the barbell across your deltoids (shoulder muscles) with

hands a little more than shoulder-width apart. Flex your hands backward, and hold your elbows high and pointed forward.

B. Assume a foot stance that's comfortable and slowly lower your body — with torso upright — into a full squat. (You can raise your heels on a 2" x 4" board to help maintain your balance.)

Return to starting position and repeat.

Cautionary Note: Be sure to hold the barbell in place securely, so that when you jump it doesn't bounce on your shoulders.

Exercise #4: BENCH SQUAT

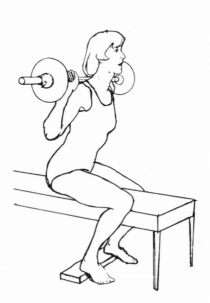
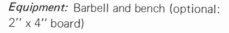
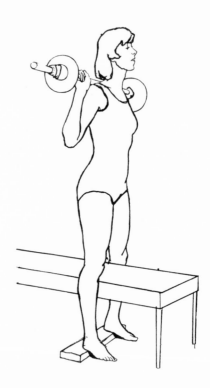

Equipment: Barbell and bench (optional: 2" x 4" board)

Muscles Worked: Excellent for thighs (quadriceps, gluteus maximus, and biceps femoris)

General Notes: You can do bench squats with the barbell held either in front or in back of your body. Doing squats on a bench is especially recommended for those people who are hesitant about going into a low position without any support because they fear knee injury.

Very heavy weights can be used, and you may very soon need a spotter and/or a rack for supporting the weight. If heavy weights are used, remember to pad the bar with a towel.

To enable yourself to gradually squat lower and lower (hence more vigorously exercising your thighs), you can start out with a higher bench, then substitute a lower and lower one.

For added comfort and better balance, you can place your heels on a 2" x 4" board.

How to Do: A. Straddle a bench (or sit on the edge of a chair) holding a barbell with a wide overgrip behind your shoulder.

B. Lower yourself into a squat until your buttocks just barely touch the bench.

Then, without sitting or resting on the bench, raise yourself and repeat — being careful to hold your torso erect throughout the movement.

Cautionary Note: It's important not to sit down on the bench at any time. You'll be using very heavy weights, and if you sit — hence relax — while you are supporting a lot of weight (especially if it's on your back), you could conceivably injure your back.

Exercise #5: JUMPING SQUAT

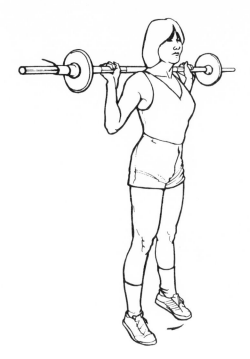

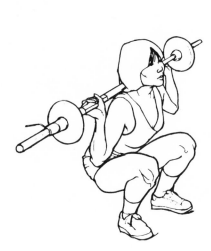

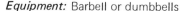

Equipment: Barbell or dumbbells

Muscles Worked: Puts better spring into thighs and calves. Exercises rectus femoris, vastus externus, and vastus internus muscles of the thighs and the gluteus medius and gluteus maximus muscles of the hips.

General Notes: This exercise is very good for building athletic strength in the thighs. It also gives your calves a good workout. Although it's normally done with a barbell held behind your neck, you can achieve about the same effects by holding a dumbbell in each hand. Relatively light weights are used for these particular squats.

How to Do: With the barbell held behind your neck (or dumbbells at your side), stand erect, with your feet pointed slightly outward and a comfortable distance apart. Hold the barbell securely in place with a wide overgrip. A. Lower yourself into a full squat, going as low as you can without losing your balance.

B. Then quickly jump up into the air as high as you can, landing in your erect starting position.

Cautionary Note: Be sure to hold the barbell in place securely, so that when you jump it doesn't bounce on your shoulders.

Exercise #6: LEG EXTENSION

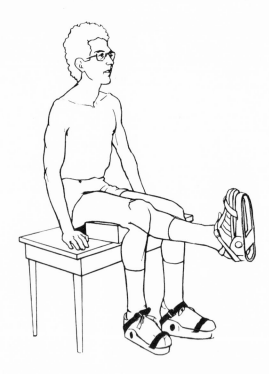

Equipment: Iron boots, bench, and a book

Muscles Worked: Front muscles of the upper leg, and lower abdomen

General Notes: If your bench isn't high enough to give the iron boots clearance, you should tuck a book under the thigh being worked. You can also do this sitting on a chair.

How to Do: A. Sitting erect on the edge of a high bench (or with the appropriate thigh, propped up on a book) and wearing the iron boots,

B. slowly raise your left leg until it is paralled with the floor. Do ten repetitions with your left leg, then switch to your right.

You can also, if you wish and if your bench is high enough, exercise both legs simultaneously. Just keep your balance by holding on to the edge of the bench.

Exercise #7: FRONT LEG RAISE

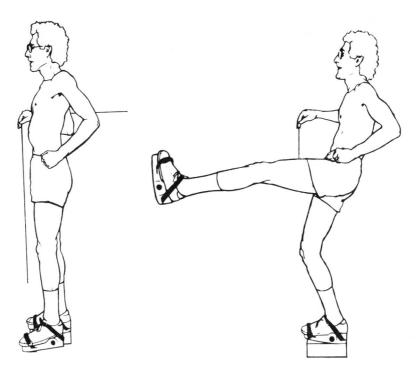

Equipment Needed: Iron boots and 2'' x 4'' block

Muscles Worked: Quadriceps, hip flexors, and lower abdomen

General Notes: This exercise builds contractile power and muscle tone in thighs. It's very good for rehabilitating knee injuries.

How to Do: A. Stand with feet together, supporting yourself with one hand on a door, wall, or piece of furniture.

B. Slowly raise the left leg until it's parallel with the ground (or higher, if you can). Do **not** swing or kick your leg up (this isn't a chorus line job). Do ten with your left leg, then ten with your right.

Exercise #8: SIDE LEG RAISE

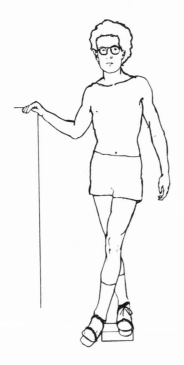 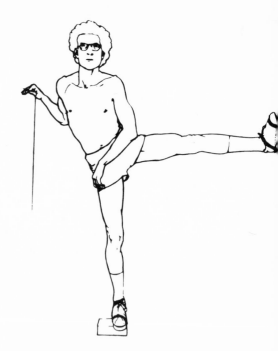

Equipment: Iron boots and 2" x 4" block

Muscles Worked: Thighs and outer muscles of the upper leg

General Notes: You should stand on a block with the foot not being exercised to give yourself a longer range of motion. Also, you should hold on to a door or something solid for balance while doing this exercise.

How to Do: A. Wearing iron boots and standing with your right foot on the left side of the block and your right leg crisscrossed over your left knee,

B. raise your right leg as high as you can without bending it. It should be parallel with the floor. Be careful not to swing or kick it up. Do ten repetitions on the right side, then switch to the left.

Exercise #9: LEG SPREAD

Exercise #10: LEG CURL

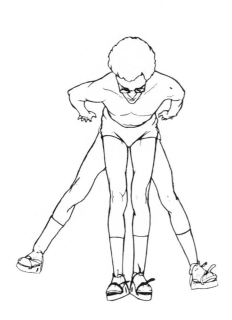

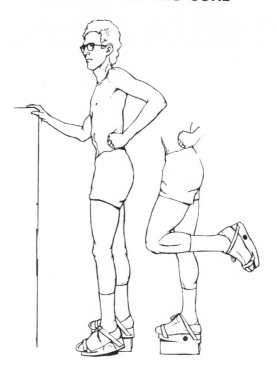

Equipment: Iron boots (optional: exercise mat or rug)

Muscles Worked: Thighs

General Notes: This is an excellent exercise for firming inner thighs.

How to Do: A. Wearing the iron boots, lie down (on an exercise mat or rug) with your legs together, straight up in the air.

B. With your hands bracing you at your sides, slowly spread your legs as far as they can go before bringing them back (slowly) to the starting position.

If you're doing this exercise correctly, you should be able to feel the stress in your thighs.

Equipment: Iron boots and something to elevate yourself off the floor (a wood block, a bench, or a book)

Muscles Worked: Hamstrings on back of upper legs

General Notes: To maintain balance while you're doing this exercise, hold on to something (a door, the wall, a piece of furniture). Also, to give the iron boot clearance as you're lifting and returning your leg, stand elevated from the floor.

The height of the bench (or chair) used helps to determine the difficulty of the exercise: one about 18" high should give you a good workout. If you wish, you can increase the difficulty by substituting a higher bench as you progress.

Exercise #11: LUNGE

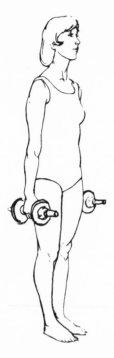

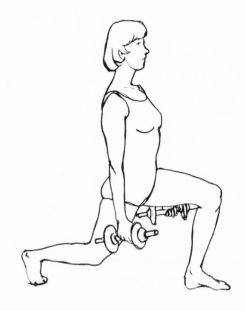

Equipment: Dumbbells or barbell

Muscles Worked: Thighs and hips

General Notes: This is hailed as being the best leg exercise for women, since it works both thighs and hips so well. (It's also great for men who are concerned about those areas of the body.) A barbell can be held behind your shoulders, or you can hold a dumbbell in each hand.

How to Do: A. Holding the weight(s) you've chosen and with your feet a comfortable distance apart, step forward with your left foot.

B. Extend it as far as you can. At the same time, lower your body until your right knee almost touches the floor and your right foot is up on its toes. Keep your head up and your torso straight.

Recover by bringing your left foot back (so that it's parallel with your right one), simultaneously returning to a standing upright position.

Exercise #12: STEP-UP

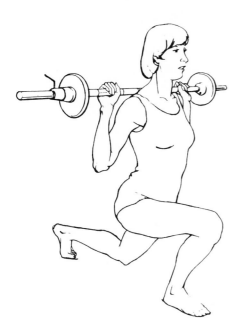 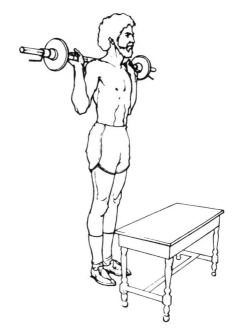

C. This exercise can be done with a barbell, extending either leg.

Then repeat the entire movement, only stepping forward this time with your right foot.

To make sure you're getting the most out of this exercise, check to make sure that your front knee extends well beyond your back of your foot when you are lunging.

Equipment: Barbell or dumbbells, and bench

Muscles Worked: Increases leg spring. Works rectus fermoris, vastus externus, and vastus internus muscles of the thighs and the gluteus medius and gluteus maximus muscles of the hips.

General Notes: This exercise can be done with a barbell, a single dumbbell, or a pair of dumbbells. Vertical and horizontal jumpers may find this exercise very helpful for increasing leg spring.

How to Do: A. Wearing th iron boots and standing erect, with hands and feet appropriately propped,

B. curl your left leg backward. Repeat this as many times as required for a set. Then do the same motion with your right leg.

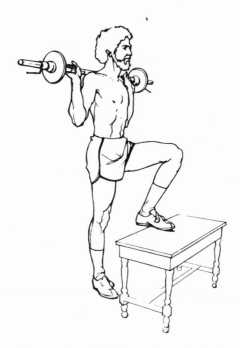

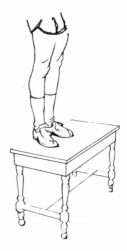

How to Do: A. When using a barbell, place it behind your neck, with hands in an overgrip wider than shoulder-width apart. (If using one or two dumbbell(s), simply hold the weight(s) comfortably in one or both hand(s).

B. Slowly step up onto the bench with the left foot, then bring up your right foot, so that

C. you're now standing erect on the bench.

Step back down, being sure to keep your body straight. Then repeat the step-up motion.

Alternate leading with each foot until you've completed the desired number of repetitions with each leg.

Exercise #13: SEATED CALF EXERCISE

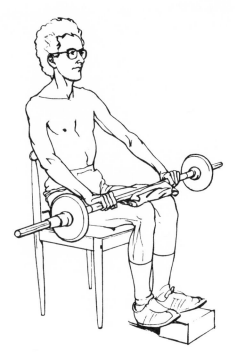

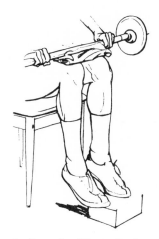

Equipment: Barbell, bench, 4"x4" block, and a towel

Muscles Worked: Swell for calves

General Notes: If using heavy weights, you should pad the bar with a towel. A high block (4"x4") makes this exercise most effective.

How to Do: A. Sit on the bench (or chair) with the barbell held in an overgrip across your knees. Use a wider-than-shoulder-width grip. Your toes should be balanced on the block placed directly in front of you on the floor.

B. Sitting up straight, slowly raise both heels up . . . then slowly lower them.

Return to starting position and repeat.

Exercise #14: DUMBBELL CALF RAISE

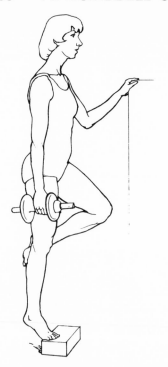
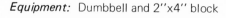
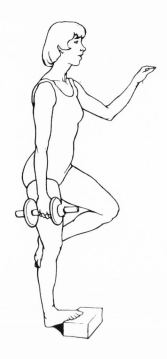

Equipment: Dumbbell and 2''x4'' block

Msucles Worked: Excellent for the calves

General Notes: This is ver effective for developing the calves, and high repetitions can be performed. Standing with your toes on a block will make this a more effective workout.

How to Do: For balance purposes, prop your free hand against something (a door, wall, piece of furniture).

A. Holding a dumbbell in your right hand and standing with your right foot's toes elevated on a block (and your left leg propped up behind your right knee), rise up and

B. down on your toes ten times. Do ten of these with'your feet pointed out (heels in), then twenty with your feet pointed straight ahead.

Switch to your left side, and repeat the same motions.

Exercise #15: BARBELL CALF RAISE

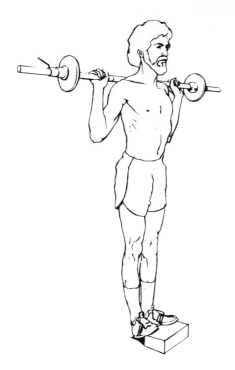
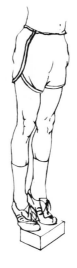

Equipment: Barbell and a 2"x4" block

Muscles Worked: Improves balance and strengthens calves. Works gastrocnemius and peroenus longus muscles of the leg and the longitudinal muscles of the feet.

General Notes: Doing this exercise on a 2"x4" block makes it more effective. You can substitute a pair of thick barbell weight plates or a book if you don't have a block handy.

How to Do: A. Stand erect with your feet together, and toes elevated on the block of wood. Hold the barbell in an overgrip across the back of your shoulders. Your hands should be more than shoulder-width apart, perhaps even as far apart as the weights allow (if this is more comfortable).

B. Slowly raise your body until you are on the toes and balls of your feet, standing soley on the block of wood. Then lower your heels back to the floor.

Exercise #16: STRADDLE HOP

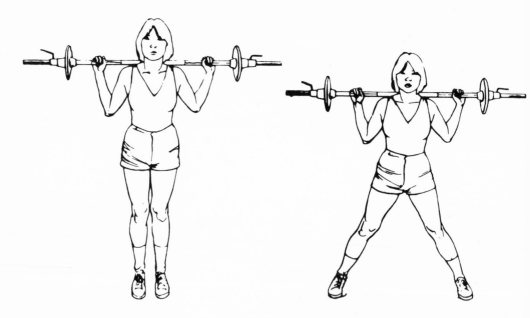

Equipment: Barbell

Muscles Worked: Builds athletic spring into calf and thigh muscles. Works thighs, legs, and the longitudinal muscles of your feet.

General Notes: This is a variation on the "jumping jacks" exercise most people have done sometime in their lives. The difference is you use a barbell while doing the jumping motion.

How to Do: A. Hold the barbell securely behind your shoulders in an overgrip. Your hands should be as far apart as possible.

B. With your feet placed closer together than shoulder-width, spring up and down while spreading your legs approximately 18" to 2' apart.

One repetition consists of hopping and spreading legs apart, then hopping and bringing legs back together.

Back Exercises

The back can be divided into three areas: the upper back (which includes the *trapezius* muscles), the middle back (which includes the *latissimus dorsi*), and the lumbar group of the lower back (consisting of the *erector spinae*).

Back exercises given here include:

17. Power Clean
18. Power Snatch
19. Upright Rowing
20. Shoulder Shrug
21. Bent Arm Pullover
22. Straight Arm Pullover
23. Bentover Rowing
24. Deadlift
25. Stiff-Leg Deadlift
26. Good Morning

Exercise #17: POWER CLEAN

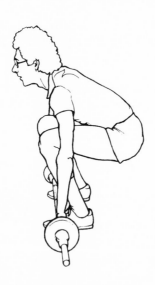

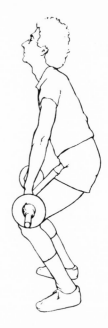

Equipment: Barbell

Muscles Worked: Virtually every muscle in the body, especially thighs, hip extensors, lumbar group of lower back, trapezius of upper back, biceps, and grip muscles.

General Notes: This involves explosive movement of the body. This means you flip the weight into the air. The power clean is particularly good for anyone who competes in sports that require explosive power, e.g., football, crew, basketball, shotput, etc.

How to Do: A. With the weight on the floor and the bar almost touching your shins, take hold of the barbell with a slightly wider-than-shoulder-width overgrip. You should pull it back towards your center of gravity. Be sure to keep your head up and your back straight (do not bow your back). Also, your hips should be low and your arms completely extended.

B. Straighten you legs, keeping your back in approximately the same angle. Your arms should still be locked until after the bar passes your knees. The barbell is actually being lifted by your legs.

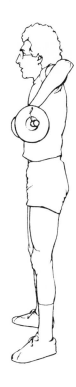

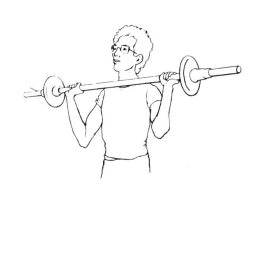

C. As soon as your legs and back are straight, your arms should follow through by pulling up the weight. Your elbows sould be up and out to the side.

D. Whip your elbows forward to cradle the bar at the base of your neck.

You have just completed the first part of the clean and press (see page 50)

Cautionary Note: This exercise involves a rather precise movement, one which you do not want to execute incorrectly. If possible, get your form checked out by. an experienced weight-trainer to make sure you're getting off to a good start with this one.

Exercise #18: POWER SNATCH

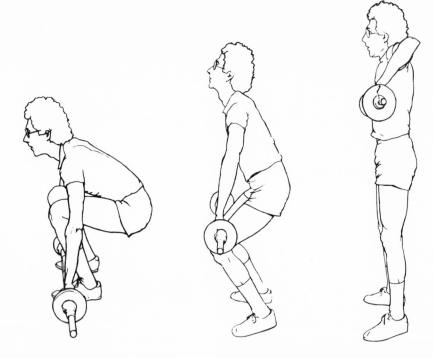

Equipment: Barbell

Muscles Worked: All the muscles in the body, including thighs, hip extensors, lumbar group of lower back, trapezius of upper back, biceps, and grip muscles.

General Notes: This exercise has very much the same effect as the power clean. It works the same muscles and uses most of the same movement. It too is very good for people who need explosive power. Because you throw the weight higher in this exercise, you should expect to do 60-70% of the weight that you can do with the power clean.

How to Do: A. With the weight on the floor and the bar almost touching your shins, take hold of the barbell with a wider overgrip (6-12" wider than for the power clean). You should pull it back towards your center of gravity. Be sure to keep your head up and your back straight (do not bow your back). Also, your hips should be low and your arms completely extended.

B. Straighten your legs, keeping your back in approximately the same angle. Your arms should remain locked until after the bar passes your knees. The barbell is actually being lifted by your legs.

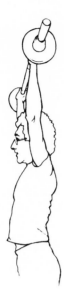

C. As soon as your legs and back are straight, your arms should follow through by pulling up the weight. Your elbows should be up and out to the side.

D. Flip the weight all the way up to locked arms' length overhead.

Reverse these steps for recovery, and repeat.

Exercise #19: UPRIGHT ROWING

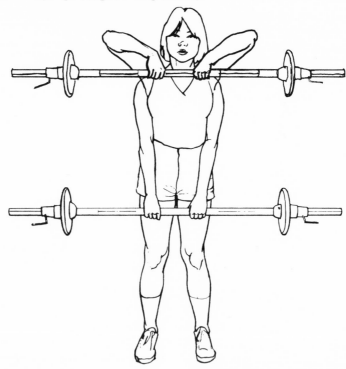

Equipment: Barbell

Muscles Worked: Trapezius and shoulder muscles

General Notes: To get maximum benefit from this exercise, there are certain things to watch for: 1) that you slowly raise the barbell . . . and *just as slowly lower it* (this is a great way to develop strength); 2) that you keep your elbows higher than your hands while doing the exercise; and 3) that you move only your arms and shoulders while doing it.

How to Do: A. Hold the center of the barbell with a narrow overgrip (about 6″) at your thighs. Your palms should be faced towards your body, and your feet in a comfortable stance, toes pointed slightly out.

B. In a slow, smooth motion raise the barbell to the base of your neck, making sure that your elbows are held high.

Then lower the barbell, resisting the weight on the way down.

Exercise #20: SHOULDER SHRUG

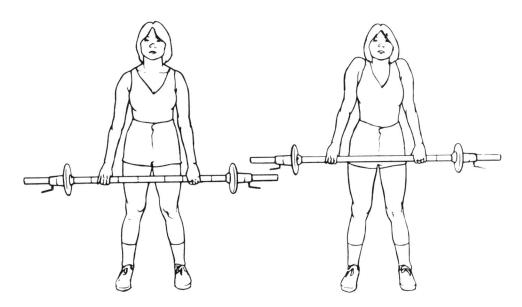

Equipment: Barbell or dumbells

Muscles Worked: Trapezius muscle of the upper back and neck, and shoulder muscles

General Notes: This has been called the most direct exercise for trapezius development. You can use either a barbell or a pair of dumbbells. In either case, your arms are nonfunctional, except to support the weight(s) so they can be suspended from your shoulders. One thing to imagine while you're doing this, in order to get the full range of motion, is to pretend that you're trying to touch your deltoids to your ears.

How to Do: A. Hold the barbell with an overgrip across the front of your thighs. Your hands should be a little more than shoulder-width apart. (Or hold dumbbells at your sides, palms pointed inward — see illustration C.)

B., C. Tighten your hands, forearms, and upper arms — rigidly aligning them. Now shrug: lower your shoulders as much as you can into a sag, then rotate them back up to as high a position as possible.

Return to your erect starting position.

Exercise #21: BENT ARM PULLOVER

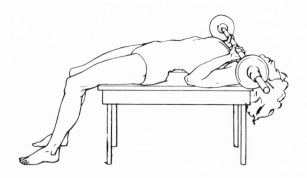
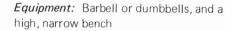
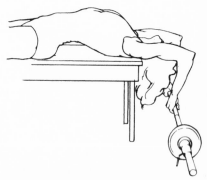

Equipment: Barbell or dumbbells, and a high, narrow bench

Muscles Worked: Middle back and chest. Also works triceps of upper arms and deltoid muscles of the shoulders.

General Notes: This exercise can be done with a barbell, a pair of dumbbells, or a single dumbbell.

How to Do: A. Lie down on a high, narrow bench, with your feet touching the floor and your head hanging over the edge of the bench. Using a narrow over-grip, hold the barbell (or dumbbells) so that it (they) rest on your chest.

B. Keeping your hands in this bent arms position, slowly lower the barbell or dumbbell(s) in a semicircle back over your head. You should get the weight as close to the floor as possible.

Slowly pull the weight back over your head to the starting position, keeping your elbows in and close together during recovery.

Exercise #22: STRAIGHT ARM PULLOVER

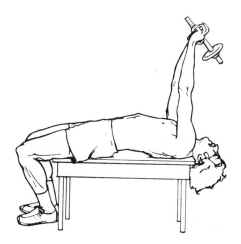
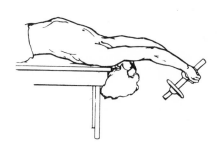

Equipment: Barbell or dumbbell(s), and bench

Muscles Worked: Good for middle back development and rib cage expansion. Works chest muscles, deltoid muscles of the shoulders, and increases chest cavity size.

General Notes: This exercise can be done with a barbell, a pair of dumbbells or a single dumbbell held in both hands. Although it's best to do this while lying on a bench, if you don't have one handy, you can lie on the floor and perform the exercise.

How to Do: A. Lying down on a bench, with your head extending over the edge and your feet planted on the floor, hold the weight with a comfortable overgrip directly over your chest, with your arms locked.

B. Slowly lower the weight in a semi-circle back over your head. Try to get the weight as close to the floor as possible. (The disadvantage of doing this on the floor is that you can lower the weight no farther than the floor.)

Return the weight along the same plane of movement back over your head and hold it stiffly above your chest. Then repeat the entire exercise.

Exercise #23: BENTOVER ROWING

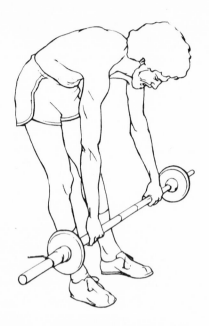
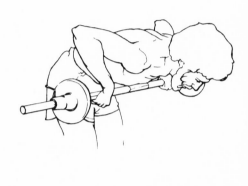

Equipment: Barbell or dumbbell(s), and bench

Muscles Worked: Latissimus dorsi muscles of the back, deltoid muscles of the shoulders, and biceps of upper arms

General Notes: This exercise can be done in several ways: you can use a barbell, two dumbbells, or you can alternate — using one dumbbell at a time.

How to Do: A. Holding a barbell with an overgrip that suits you (probably greater than shoulder-width), place your feet comfortably apart and bend your knees slightly, then bend over. The weight should almost be touching the ground.

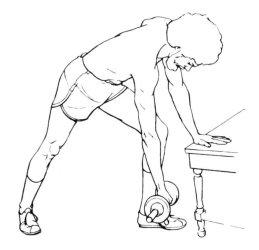 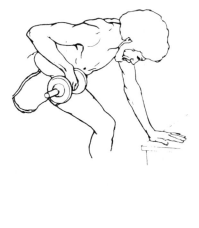

B. With your arms hanging perpendicular to your torso, slowly pull the weight up to your chest. Then slowly lower it back to the starting position.

C. If exercising one arm at a time with a single dumbbell, you can lean forward and, with the leg of the exercising side straight back, support your body with your free hand.

The advantage to using one dumbbell to do this exercise is that you can work your upper back without putting any stress on your lower back (since you're supporting your body with one hand).

Exercise #24: DEADLIFT

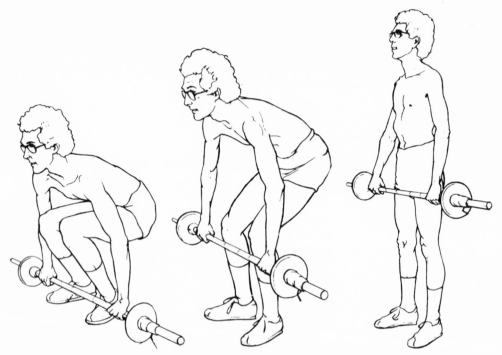

Equipment: Barbell

Muscles Worked: Develops lower back, works thigh muscles and hips.

General Notes: Very heavy weights can be used in this exercise. A special lifting belt can be worn to give additional support to your body when you reach an advanced stage. Also, with heavy weights you should use a mixed grip — one hand in an overgrip and the other in an under-grip. (This is to insure that the bar doesn't slip out of your fingers.) According to Bill Reynolds, trained male lifters can do almost 900 lbs. in this exercise. But don't try that for a while . . .

How to Do: A. With the barbell lying on the floor in front of you, almost against your shins, stand in a half-squatting position. Your feet should be comfortably apart, and you should use a slightly wider-than-shoulder-width overgrip.

B. Slowly pull the weight and begin to straighten your body.

C. Keep pulling up on the weight until you are standing erect with the barbell held as high across your thighs as possible — without bending your arms.

Recovery involves slowly lowering your body while holding the barbell without bending your arms, and returning to your starting position, where you are in a half-squat and the barbell is on the floor.

Exercise #25: STIFF-LEG DEADLIFT

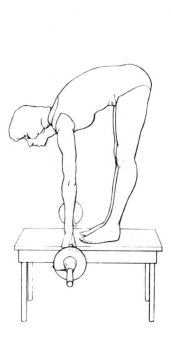

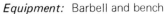

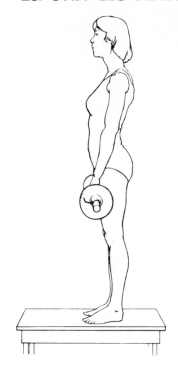

Equipment: Barbell and bench

Muscles Worked: Lumbar muscles of the lower back and the thigh biceps (hamstrings)

General Notes: It's best to do this while standing on a bench. This is to give you a wider range of movement, so that the barbell plates don't touch the floor and prevent you from stretching as far as you might.

How to Do: A. Standing on a bench and holding a barbell with an overgrip slightly wider than shoulder-width,

B. slowly bend over, being sure to keep your back flat and your hands, forearms, and upper arms locked in a straight line. Your back should become slightly arched as you lower the barbell to the bench.

Then slowly return your body to an erect position, with your back slightly arched. The bar should reach its highest position on your thighs. Be sure not to bend your legs or arms while doing this exercise.

Exercise #26: GOOD MORNING

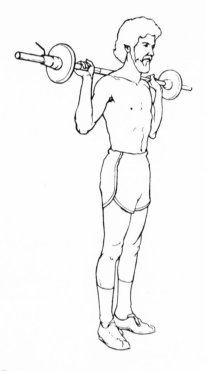

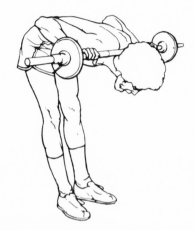

Equipment: Barbell

Muscles Worked: Lower back and thigh biceps

General Notes: If doing this exercise with legs locked, you should use a relatively light weight. Some people prefer to do it with heavier weights and legs unlocked. This exercise has much the same effect as the stiff-leg deadlift.

How to Do: A. Stand erect with your feet locked out, holding the barbell across the back of your shoulders. Use an overgrip that spaces your hands a comfortable distance apart.

B. Bend over as far as you can, without bending your legs (if using light weights). If using heavy weights, bend your knees slightly.

Return to starting position.

Chest Exercises

The chest consists of pectoral muscles, made up of two groups (the *pectoralis minor* (the smaller upper pectoral) and the *pectoralis major* (the larger lower pectoral).

Chest exercises include:

27. Bench Press
28. Lying Straight Arm Lateral
29. Lying Bent Arm Lateral

Exercise #27: BENCH PRESS

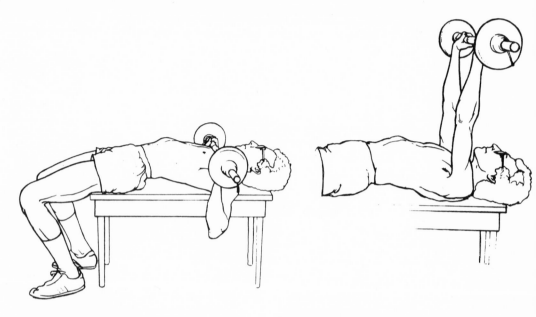

Equipment: Barbell or dumbbells, and bench

Muscles Worked: Entire pectoral area, triceps of upper arms, and deltoids of shoulders

General Notes: This is one of the exercises that come into mind immediately when you mention weight-training. It works the entire pectoral area very effectively and is considered by many experts to be the best upper-body exercise.

How far apart you place your hands on the barbell will give you different results. It's recommended to start out with a greater-than-shoulder-width overgrip, then to graduate to more difficult positions.

If using dumbbells instead of a barbell, hold them vertically or parallel to your chest.

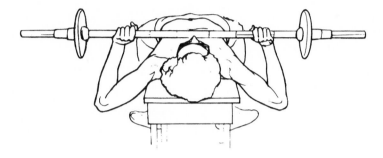

How to Do: A. Lie back on a bench, holding the barbell with an overgrip.

B. Then push the weight straight up over your head without bending your arms.

C. Lower the barbell straight down until it touches your mid-chest.

Then repeat steps B & C for as many repetitions as your program requires.

Cautionary Note: You should use a weight rack to support the barbell when you advance to heavier weights. If you don't have a rack, have a person who can help you get the weight on and off your chest.

Exercise #28: LYING STRAIGHT ARM LATERAL

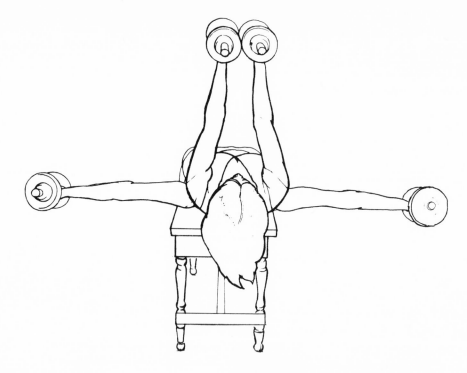

Equipment: Dumbbells

Muscles Worked: Pectorals

General Notes: To make this exercise more difficult and to work different parts of your pectorals, perform it on an inclined or a declined bench. You can also do it on the floor, if you don't have a flat bench, but you won't get the full range of motion since the dumbbell plates will hit the floor.

How to Do: A. Lying down, hold the dumbbells above your chest at arms' length. The dumbbells should be touching each other.

B. Being sure to keep your arms straight and locked, slowly lower the dumbbells to your sides. If lying on a bench, let the dumbbells get as close to the floor as possible.

Then with arms still locked, return to starting position and repeat.

Cautionary Note: If you feel strain on the inside of your elbows while doing this exercise with your arms locked, you might prefer doing the Lying Bent Arm Lateral (see next exercise).

Exercise #29: LYING BENT ARM LATERAL

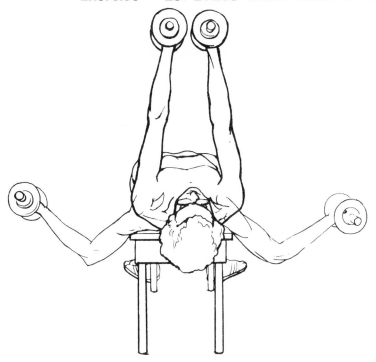

Equipment: Dumbbells and bench

Muscles Worked: Pectorals

General Notes: This, like the lying straight arm lateral, can be done on the floor or a flat bench. It may be a little easier to do than the straight arm version since your arms are allowed to bend. And more weight can be used.

How to Do: A. Lie down. the dumbbells held arm's length above your chest.

B. Slightly bending your elbows, slowly bring the weights down to your sides as far as you can go.

Return to starting position, and repeat.

Shoulder Exercises

Developing your deltoid muscles in your shoulders will be valuable in all physical activities, from everyday chores to performance in sports. The deltoids can be divided into three sections, or heads: 1) the *anterior head,* which moves the arm forward; 2) the *medial head* (side), which moves the arm sideways; and 3) the *posterior head* (rear), which helps the arm move backwards.

Shoulder exercises also affect the chest. Included here are:

30. Military Press
31. Press behind Neck
32. Front Lateral Raise
33. Side Lateral Raise
34. Bentover Lateral

Exercise #30: MILITARY PRESS

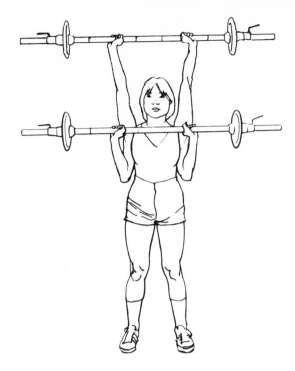

Equipment: Barbell

Muscles Worked: Triceps of the upper arms and the deltoids of the shoulders. Also trapezius and upper chest.

General Notes: This is called the most basic of all shoulder exercises, and constitutes the second part of the clean & press (see page 00). You can also do military presses while seated, if you wish.

How to Do: A. Stand erect, holding a barbell with an overgrip that's about shoulder-width. The weight should be held at shoulder height. Your hands should be flexed backwards and your elbows pointed forward. You should stand comfortably, with toes pointed slightly out.

B. Slowly push the barbell upward until it's straight above your head and your arms are locked. As the barbell goes up and down, it should pass close to your face (you should hold the weight close to your body).

Return the barbell to your shoulders for recovery.

Exercise #31: PRESS BEHIND NECK

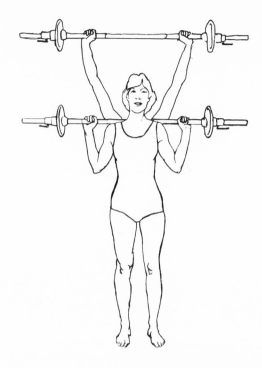

Equipment: Barbell

Muscles Worked: Triceps of upper arms and deltoids of shoulders

General Notes: Bodybuilders really like this exercise because it can quickly broaden shoulders. You can also perform this exercise while seated. Another variation is to alternate presses from the front (military presses) with these presses behind the neck.

How to Do: A. Stand erect, with your feet a comfortable distance apart. Hold the barbell on your shoulders behind your neck. Use an overgrip which has your hands about 6" more than shoulder-width apart.

B. Push the barbell up above your head until it's at arm's length.

Then lower it back to the starting position.

Exercise #32: FRONT LATERAL RAISE

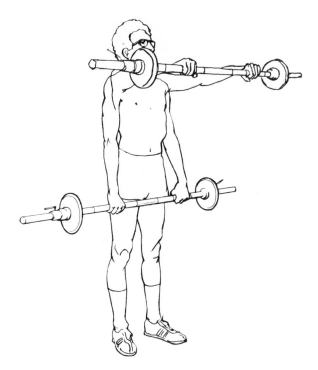

Equipment: Barbell or dumbbells

Muscles Worked: Anterior head of the deltoids

General Notes: Relatively light weights are used for this exercise. You can use a barbell, a pair of dumbbells (either simultaneously, or alternately raising one).

How to Do: A. Stand erect, holding the barbell with a shoulder-width overgrip. Your arms should be stiff, supporting the barbell across the upper thighs.

B. Being sure to keep your arms straight, slowly raise the barbell in a semicircular motion until it is arm's length over your head.

Return to starting position.

Exercise #33: SIDE LATERAL RAISE

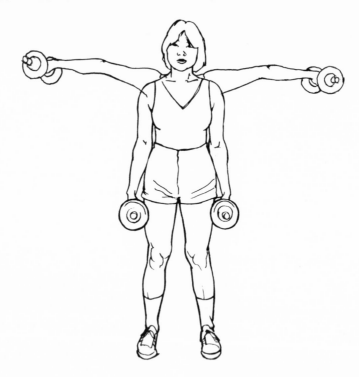

Equipment: Dumbbells

Muscles Worked: Anterior and medial deltoid head of shoulders

General Notes: How you hold the dumbbells — with palms up or down — puts stress on different parts of your deltoids. Done palms down, this exercise stresses the medial deltoid heads, while palms up affects the anterior head.

How to Do: A. Stand erect, holding a dumbbell in each hand at your sides. Your arms should be straight and locked.

B. Raise the dumbbells in a semicircle out to your sides until your upper arms are parallel to the floor or slightly higher.

Return to starting position and repeat.

Cautionary Note: When you perform this exercise with palms up, you can use considerably more weight. A relatively light weight should be used when doing the side lateral raise with palms down.

Exercise #34: BENTOVER LATERAL

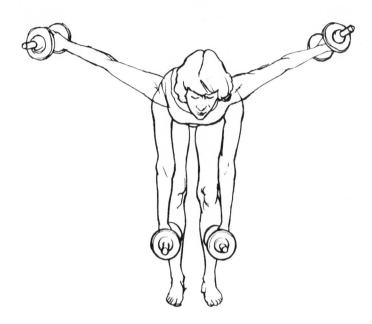

Equipment: Dumbbells

Muscles Worked: Shoulders and upper back

General Notes: It is important to maintain the same bent-over torso position throughout the movement of this exercise.

How to Do: A. Holding a dumbbell in each hand, with your feet fairly close together, bend over from the waist. Your waist should be parallel to the floor. With your legs slightly bent, hold the dumbbells directly below your chest. Your arms should be straight.

B. Bring the dumbbells straight out to your sides until they're positioned above your torso. Keep your head looking down.

Return to starting position and repeat.

Upper Arm Exercises

Upper arm muscles include the biceps and the triceps. The biceps allow you to bend your arms, while the triceps help you straighten your arms. Muscles aren't totally isolated in exercises of course, and many of the exercises described in other sections also affect the biceps and triceps (e.g., military presses, bench presses, and presses behind the neck for the triceps, and upright rowing, bentover rowing for the biceps).

Upper arm exercises include:
35.   Barbell Curls
36.   Dumbbell Curls
37.   Concentration Curls
38.   Barbell French Press
39.   Dumbbell French Press
40.   Dumbbell Kickback

Exercise #35: BARBELL CURLS

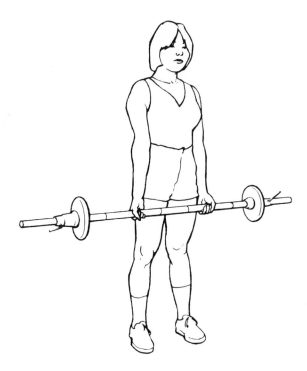

Equipment: Barbell

Muscles Worked: Biceps

General Notes: This is referred to as the basic biceps exercise. It can be done with different width grips — shoulder-width, wider, or narrower.

How to Do: A. Stand erect, with feet in a comfortable stance. Hold the barbell with an undergrip across the front of your thighs.

B. Holding your elbows against the sides of your torso, very slowly bring the barbell up in a curling motion.

C. When the bar approaches your upper chest and neck, flex your hands and continue the curling motion until it nearly touches your chin.

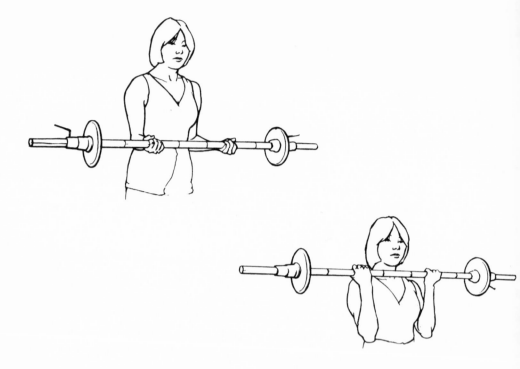

Return to starting position and repeat.

To work your biceps even more vigorously, you can do this exercise with your back held straight against a wall. This almost totally eliminates the use of your legs and upper body, so that all the work is concentrated on your biceps.

Cautionary Note: Be careful to maintain good form: don't cheat by swinging the bar up to get it started. The entire motion should be ultra-smooth, never jerky. If you keep your elbows in tight and concentrate on doing each movement with almost exaggerated slowness, you should be all right.

Exercise #36: DUMBBELL CURLS

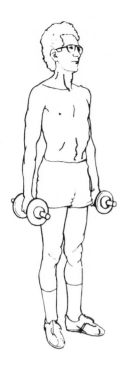

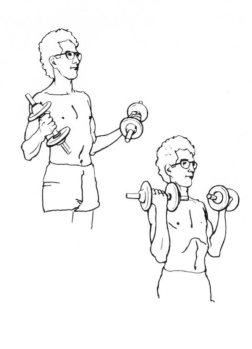

Equipment: Dumbbells

Muscles Worked: Biceps

General Notes: There are many possible versions of this exercise. You can use two dumbbells simultáneously or one at a time. Your palms can be facing forward (as though doing the barbell curl), or they can face each other. You can stand or sit while performing these curls, which require less wrist and elbow flexibility than barbell curls.

If you start out with palms forward, they should end up facing you (see illustration C). In other words, your palms rotate.

How to Do: A. Stand with dumbbells held at your side.

B. Slowly curl them up to your upper chest or chin.

C. When the dumbbells approach your upper chest, flex your hands and continue the curling action until they nearly touch your chin.

Return to starting position and repeat.

Exercise #37: CONCENTRATION CURLS

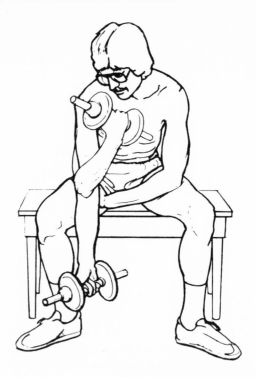

Equipment: Dumbbell and bench

Muscles Worked: Biceps

General Notes: This exercise looks like the "thinking person's" cup of tea. And, indeed, it requires a pensive mood. Only one arm is exercised at a time, with the free arm used to anchor the weight-bearing one. This is to concentrate all the work on the one particular muscle or muscle group.

How to Do: A. Sit on the edge of a bench, holding a single dumbbell in your right hand. Brace your elbow against your right inner thigh — making sure your upper arm doesn't move while you perform the exercise. Your legs should be spread apart, and your feet planted firmly on the floor.

B. With your left hand bracing your right elbow, lean forward and curl the dumbbell up to your shoulder. You should be staring at the weight as you perform the movement. If you can, twist your little finger as close to your body as possible.

Exercise #38: (BARBELL) FRENCH PRESS

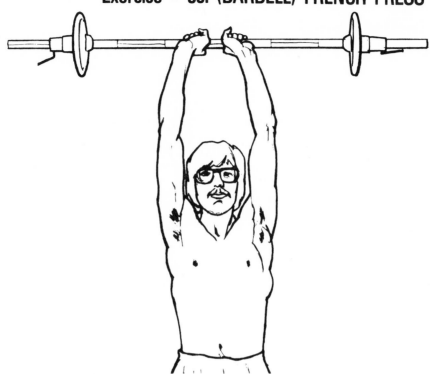

Equipment: Barbell

Muscles Worked: Triceps

General Notes: This is called the basic triceps developer. You can stand or sit while performing it.

How to Do: A. Stand erect, holding a barbell with a narrow overgrip (about 6'') over your head, with your arms extended straight up.

87

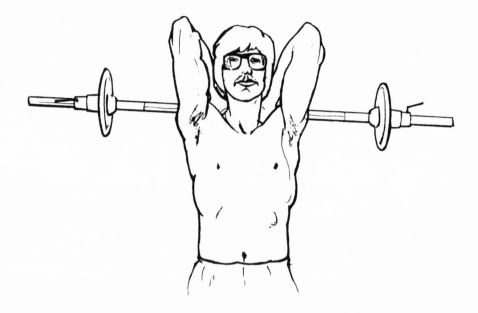

B. While your upper arms and elbows remain stationary, lower the barbell in a semicircle motion to the back of your neck. Only your forearms move. Your elbows should be pointing up when you reach the low position of the movement.

Slowly return to the starting position. If you're doing it right, you'll definitely feel the stress in your triceps.

Exercise #39: (DUMBBELL) FRENCH PRESS

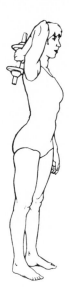
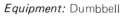

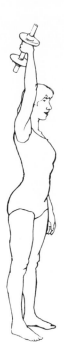

Equipment: Dumbbell

Muscles Worked: Triceps

General Notes: There are several different ways to perform this exercise. You can use one dumbbell at a time (as shown), holding it with one hand (illustrations C & D). Or, you can even hold a dumbbell in each hand, and work each arm simultaneously. This exercise can be done sitting or standing.

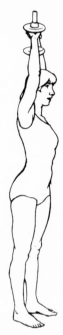

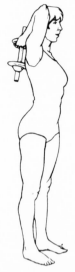

How to Do: A. Stand erect, holding a dumbbell directly over your head, extended at arm's length.

B. Slowly bring it down in a semicircle to the back of your neck, remembering to keep your upper arm and elbow stationary. Only your forearm should move.

Return to starting position and repeat.

Exercise #40: DUMBBELL KICKBACK

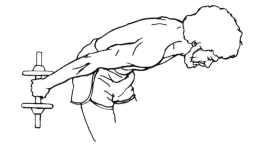

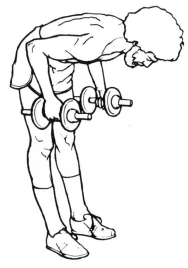

Equipment: Dumbbells

Muscles Worked: Triceps

General Notes: You can perform this exercise with either one dumbbell at a time, or with one held in each hand at the same time. If you decide to do it with only one dumbbell, place your nonexercising hand on a bench or chair to support yourself.

How to Do: A. Holding the dumbbell(s), bend forward with your exercise arm(s) held at a right angle to your body.

B. Straighten out your arm(s), until it (they) extend behind you parallel to the floor.

Return to starting position and repeat.

Forearm Exercises

The muscles of your lower arms are used for almost everything you do. Developing them will make life a lot easier, as well as improve your performance in many sports and physical activities in general. Forearm strength is particularly valuable for sports which involve throwing, e.g., baseball and shotputting. And, of course, it is also very good for tennis.

Forearm exercises include:

41.   Reverse Curl

42.   Wrist Curl

43.   Reverse Wrist Curl

Exercise #41: REVERSE CURL

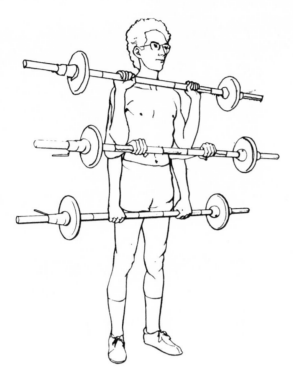

Equipment: Barbells

Muscles Worked: Extensor-flexor group muscles of the forearms, and biceps

General Notes: The width of the grip you use will place different stress on your muscles. If you wish to work your forearm muscles more vigorously, use a narrower grip than recommended below. Just be aware that you'll be able to do about 20% less weight that way.

How to Do: A. standing erect, with your feet a comfortable distance apart, hold a barbell with a shoulder-width overgrip. The barbell should be resting against your upper thighs.

B. With your hands and forearms locked in rigid alignment, slowly bring the barbell up towards your chest in a curling motion. Your elbows should be pinned to your sides.

C. Curl the bar up to your upper chest or chin.

Return to starting position and repeat.

Exercise #42: WRIST CURL

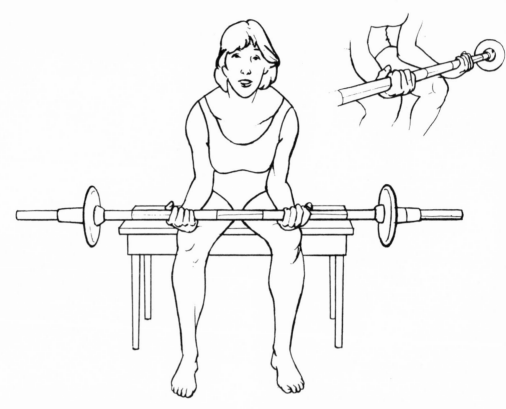

Equipment: Barbell or dumbbells, and bench

Muscles Worked: Extensor-flexor group muscles of the forearms

General Notes: You can do this exercise with a barbell, one dumbbell at a time, or two dumbbells simultaneously.

How to Do: A. While seated on a bench, legs spread apart, hold a barbell with a shoulder-width undergrip. Your forearms should be resting on your thighs, and your fists should be supported by your knees.

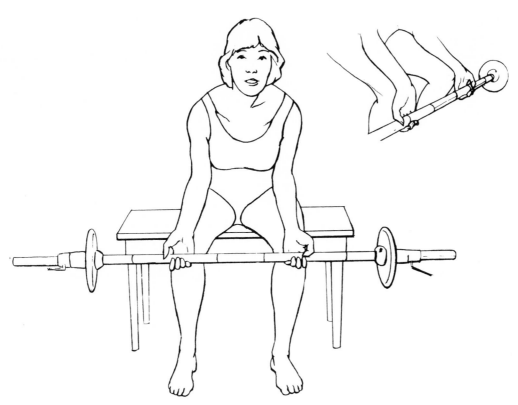

B. Slowly bend your fists down as low as they will go, to the extent of rolling the bar down your fingers.

Then curl the bar back up as high as possible, while flexing your wrists as hard as you can.

If you do this with one dumbbell at a time, you should rest your nonexercising elbow on your nonexercising side's knee, and tuck your hand under your exercising elbow.

Exercise #43: REVERSE WRIST CURL

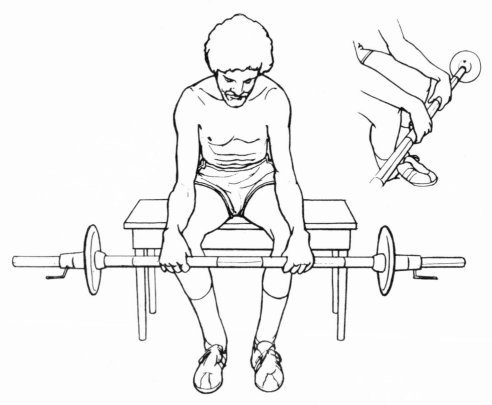

Equipment: Barbell or dumbbells, and
bench

Muscles Worked: Forearms

General Notes: As with the other curls,
there are several possible versions of this
exercise. You can perform it with a barbell, a single dumbbell, or a pair of dumbbells. You can sit and do the exercise, or
you can kneel behind a low bench while
doing it.

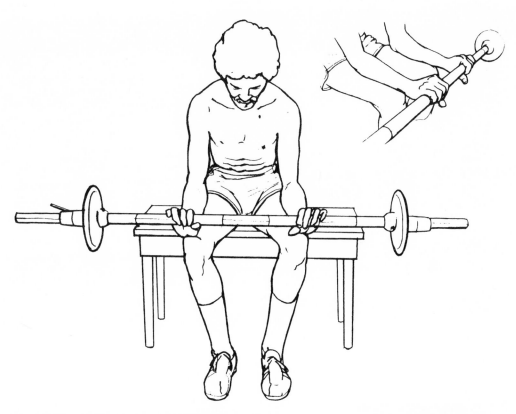

How to Do: A. Sitting on a bench, hold the barbell with a shoulder-width overgrip across the front of your legs.

B. With your elbows resting on your thighs, slowly curl the bar down as far as you can go, with palms pointed down.

Slowly return the barbell to the starting position and repeat.

Abdominal Exercises

Stronger abdominal muscles not only will improve your appearance but will help support your mid-body better. These muscles are involved in drawing up your legs for any activity. These are also the muscles that help protect your vital internal organs.

When performing abdominal exercises, you should use light weights, but in high repetitions (20-100).

Abdominal and waist exercises include:

44. Sit-up
45. Leg Raise
46. Knee-up
47. Sidebend
48. Twisting
49. Bentover Twisting

Exercise #44: SIT-UP

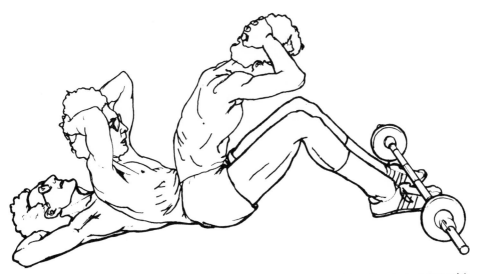

Equipment: Barbell (optional: weight plate)

Muscles Worked: Abdominal

General Notes: This is a highly effective abdominal exercise. It can be performed with or without a weight plate (see illustration D) to give added resistance. You should, however, always brace your feet under a barbell (or have someone hold your feet). Notice how your knees should be unlocked: this is to keep unnecessary strain off of your lower back.

If you do use weight plates, start out with 5 lbs. and work your way up. If you're really strong, you may be able to advance to 40 lbs. this way. But anything less than that will be quite effective.

The general rule to follow is that if you can get up to doing fifty sit-ups without any resistance, add some weight and drop your number of repetitions down to about twenty. Then work your way up, and add some more weight (in 5 lb. increments).

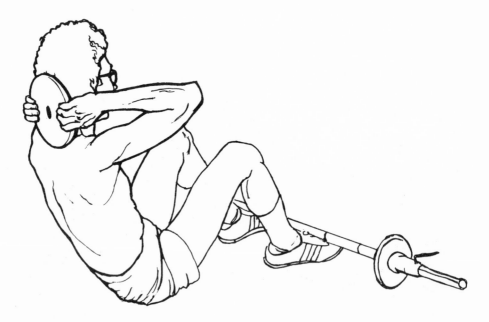

How to Do: A. Lie down on the floor with your hands laced behind your head and your legs slightly bent, with feet pinned or held.

B. Curl your body upward and forward in a semicircle.

C. Continue curling until your elbows (or head, if you want to stretch more) touch your thighs.

Be sure to keep your back arched throughout, and do not jerk your body up (having your feet braced will help prevent bad form).

To make the exercise more difficult, you can do it on an inclined board, where your legs will be higher than the rest of your body.

Exercise #45: LEG RAISE

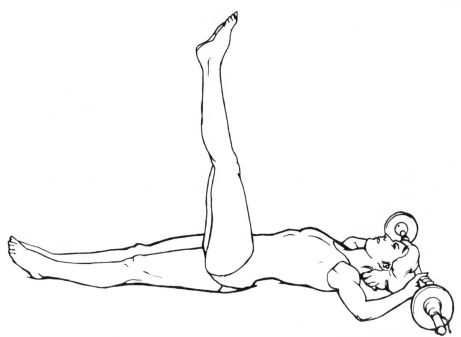

Equipment: Barbell (optional: iron boots)

Muscles Worked: Abdominal

General Notes: You can get good results from doing this exercise without any weights. But if you'd like a really tough workout for your abdomen, do it with iron boots.

How to Do: A. Lie down on the floor, hanging on to a barbell above your head. (Or place your hands by your hips so that your arms and upper body won't move.)

B. With your legs almost locked, raise them up slowly until they are perpendicular to your torso.

C. If you really want to push it, continue to raise your legs until your ankles touch your head.

Return legs slowly to starting position, and repeat.

Exercise #46: KNEE-UP

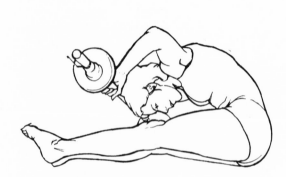

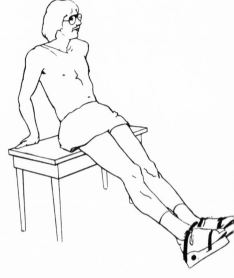

Cautionary Note: Be sure to avoid jerking your legs up and down. If you jerk you won't be working the proper muscles.

Equipment: Bench (optional: iron boots)

Muscles Worked: Abdominal

General Notes: This is one of the milder abdominal exercises, so it's best to do it with iron boots to give yourself a tougher workout.

How to Do: A. Wearing the iron boots, sit on the edge of a low bench (or chair). Lean back, bracing your upper body with your hands holding on to the sides of the bench (or chair). Extend your legs so that they're straight out ahead of you, with feet touching the floor.

Exercise #47: SIDEBEND

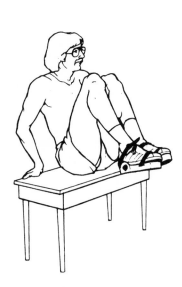

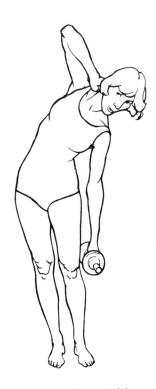

B. Pull your knees up to your chest; your knees should end up pointing at your head.

Return to starting position by thrusting your legs back down and out straight. Your feet shouldn't touch the floor again until you rest.

Equipment: Barbell or dumbbell(s)

Muscles Worked: External oblique muscles at the sides of your waist

General Notes: Light weights and high repetitions should be used when doing this exercise to prevent building up the side muscles (which would make your waist look bigger).

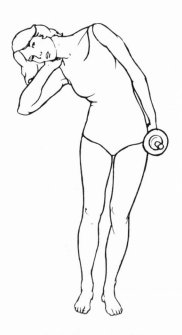

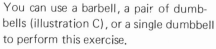

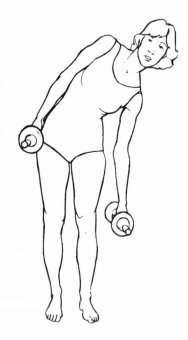

You can use a barbell, a pair of dumb-bells (illustration C), or a single dumbbell to perform this exercise.

How to Do: A. Holding a single dumb-bell in your left hand, place your right hand on the side of your neck. Bend down to your left side as far as possible.

B. Return to erect position, then bend down to your right side. Try to get your hand (holding the dumbbell) as close to your foot as possible.

Your head should be tilted down, as if a string were attaching it to your foot and your head were being pulled (like a puppet).

If using a barbell, hold it in place with a very wide overgrip across your shoulders behind your neck. Your feet should be shoulder-width apart.

Exercise #48: TWISTING

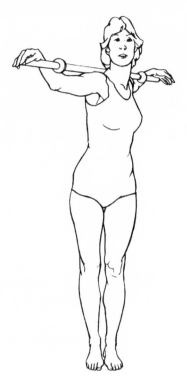

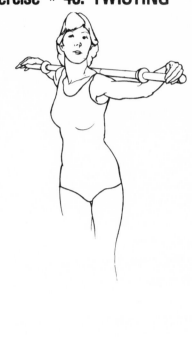

Equipment: Bar (no weights)

Muscles Worked: This is good for trimming your waist, as well as for increasing lower back flexibility.

General Notes: You can do this either standing or seated, straddling a bench. If it's hard for you to keep your hips from twisting along with the rest of your body, it may be better for you to perform this exercise seated on a bench.

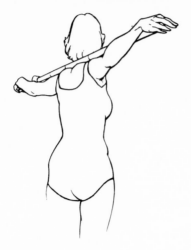

How to Do: A. Stand up with your feet together and wrap your arms around an unloaded bar held behind your neck. Twist your torso to one side.

B. Then twist to the opposite side.

For this exercise to work effectively on your waist it's important not to move your hips.

Exercise #49: BENTOVER TWISTING

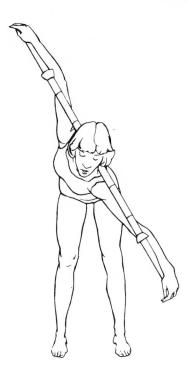
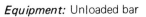
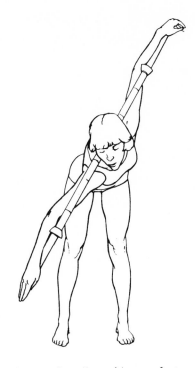

Equipment: Unloaded bar

Muscles Worked: External obliques of waist

General Notes: This is a waist-slimmer. It also increases lower back flexibility.

How to Do: A. Standing with your feet wide apart, wrap your arms around an unloaded bar held behind your neck. Bend over and twist to one side.

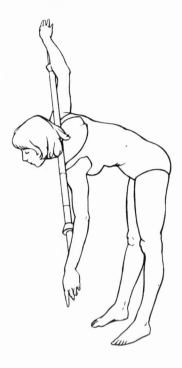

B. Return to erect position; then bend
over and twist to opposite side.

Neck Exercises

Having strong neck muscles is something most people don't think about, but they are important in such sports as wrestling and football. More important, neck strength can make a big difference if you're involved in an accident or injury that involves your neck.

Two exercises for the neck are given here:

50. Wrestler's Bridge
51. Self Hand Pressure

Exercise #50: WRESTLER'S BRIDGE

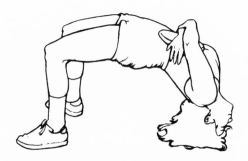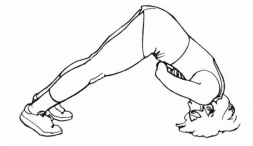

Equipment: Optional: weight plate

Muscles Worked: Neck and upper back

General Notes: This exercise is aptly named, since it's based on a critical move-ment for wrestlers. It's a very effective exercise to strengthen and develop all the muscles of your neck.

How to Do: A. Lie down on your back on an exercise mat or rug and raise your body so that only your head and feet are touching the ground. Holding a weight plate across your chest (or simply placing your hands there), rock forward and back-ward. Then from side to side.

B. You can also do this with your head and chest pointed down. In this case, you can place your hands either behind your back (using no weight plate) or in front, across your chest. Rock forward and back-ward, then from side to side.

Exercise #51: SELF HAND PRESSURE

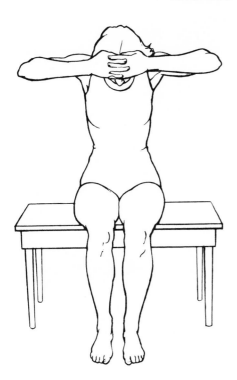
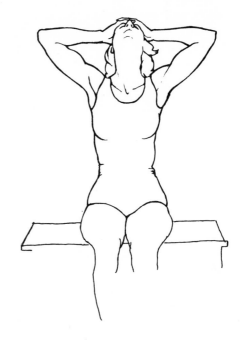

Equipment: Bench or chair

Muscles Worked: Neck

General Notes: This is an exercise that's easy to perform almost anywhere (you can do it at work, at school, while watching TV). It requires no equipment or training partner. All you need are your own hands to apply pressure to various parts of your head to work various neck muscles.

How to Do: A. Sitting on a bench or chair (or even on the floor), place your hands on top of your head, lacing your fingers together. Apply pressure as you bring your head up and down.

B. You can do the same thing with your hands applied to the side of your head or with your hands placed behind your neck.

Stretching Exercises

There are many stretching exercises that are used by coaches, dance instructors, athletes, practitioners of yoga, and anyone else interested in increasing flexibility. We've already talked about the importance of stretching to weight-training. So take your pick of the following and add them to any repertoire of stretching exercises you may already have:

LEG LIFT: Standing erect, with legs slightly apart, and stomach held in, lift your left leg (don't kick it up) and hold it as high and as straight as you can. Do not bend your knee. Be sure your torso is straight and that you're not slumping or jerking. Hold your leg up there for a count of three. Do ten of these on your left side; then repeat with your right leg. To help improve your balance, don't hang on to anything for support. Pretend you're a ballet dancer — this might help you feel more graceful and confident.

ARM CIRCLES: Standing erect, with legs slightly apart, hold your arms straight out (they should be parallel to the floor, as though you were ready to fly). Rotate your arms in a complete circle . . . first backwards, then forwards. This warms up your arm joints. Do ten in one direction; then reverse. Be sure to execute the movement slowly and rhythmically.

HEAD ROTATION: Standing erect (or sitting, if you prefer), pretend you're an Afro jazz dancer and rotate your head in a complete circle — slowly. Do about ten of these going clockwise, then ten counterclockwise.

UPPER SHOULDER LOOSENER: Standing erect, with legs slightly apart, bring your left arm up, placing your left hand just under your neck. With your right arm, grasp your left upper arm above the elbow and pull gently down. This is very good for relieving tension that may be hidden in those joints. Repeat this about fifteen times.

WAIST TWIST: Standing erect, with legs shoulder-width apart, place your hands on your hips, being sure to keep your hips forward. Turn to your right side, looking behind you as you do it. Return to the starting position, then turn to your left. Your toes should be pointing forward while you perform this exercise. Do about ten for each side.

HAND WALK: Sitting on the floor or on an exercise mat with your legs comfortably apart, walk your hands to the center (in between your feet), being sure to keep your head up. The first time you do this, it should feel comfortable. The second time you do it, you should stretch a bit — just enough to make yourself feel it (but it still shouldn't be painful). Keep your hands flat on the floor — don't jerk or bounce, and hold for a count of fifteen. Then repeat the movement a half dozen times, each time stretching just a little farther, and maybe holding still a bit longer.

CHEST-TO-FLOOR: In the same position as above, grab one ankle with both hands, being sure to keep your head up. Try to get your entire chest to touch your thigh, and your elbows to touch the ground. Start with the right side, then the left. Next try to extend your chest to the center of your legs, getting your chest to touch the ground.

HIP FLEXOR: Standing erect, with legs slightly apart, pull your right leg up from behind with your right hand. Do this ten times, then repeat the motion with your left leg and hand.

These are just a few possibilities. Do as many of them as you like, but be sure to do at least a few stretching movements before each weight-training workout and on your "rest days." The idea is to get loose and flexible and to make your entire body feel more comfortable with vigorous physical activity.

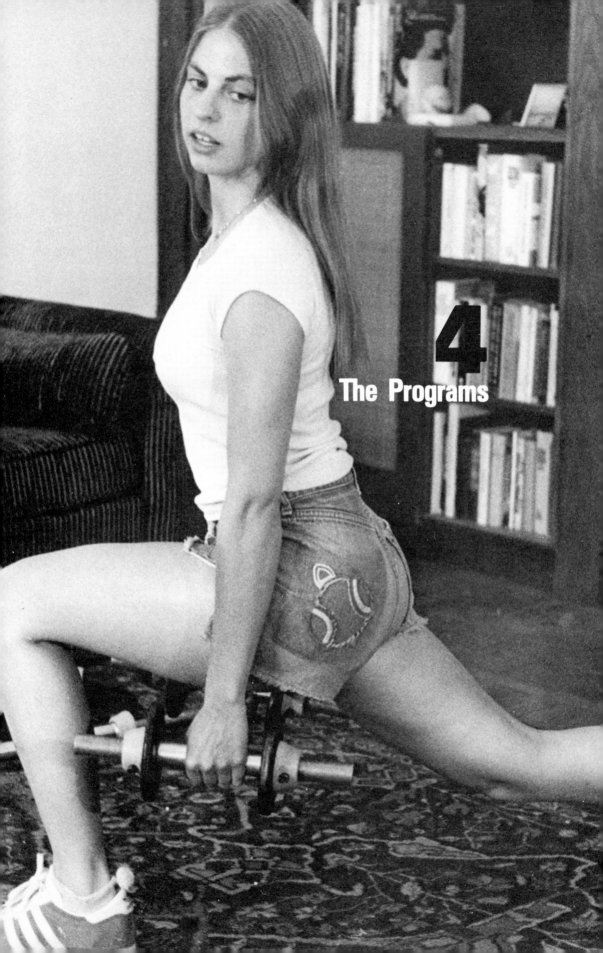

4

The Programs

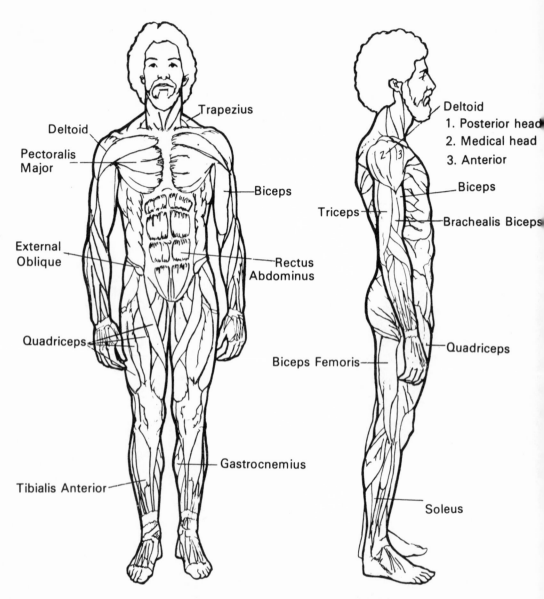

Trapezius

Deltoid

Pectoralis
Major

Biceps

External
Oblique

Rectus
Abdominus

Quadriceps

Biceps Femoris

Gastrocnemius

Tibialis Anterior

Deltoid
1. Posterior head
2. Medical head
3. Anterior

Biceps

Triceps

Brachealis Biceps

Quadriceps

Soleus

These programs have been designed for general fitness and specific sports with the help of Bill Reynolds. Except for the general beginning and intermediate programs the same programs are intended for women and men. (All of the exercises, too, are suitable for both women and men. That the illustration shows a woman or man performing a particular exercise does not mean the exercise is necessarily better for a member of that sex.).

The suggested amount of weight to use for each exercise is given in terms of a percentage of *your body weight.* This percentage is the total weight used in the exercise, so if you're using dumbbells you should use half the amount suggested in each hand. Like the sets and repetitions, these percentages are only suggestions.

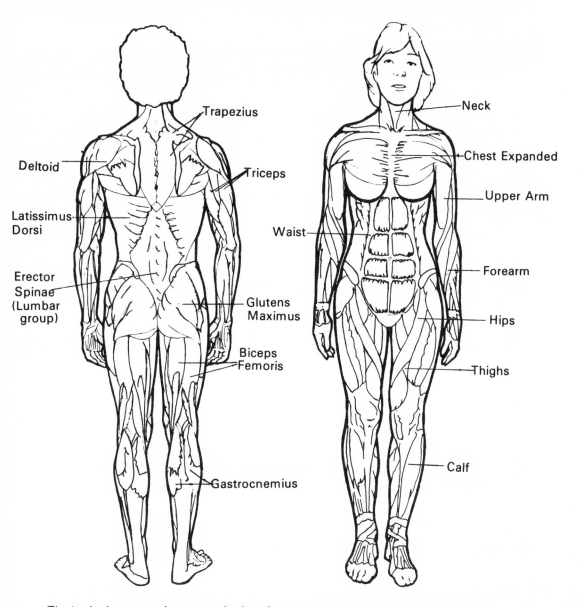

Trapezius

Deltoid

Latissimus Dorsi

Erector Spinae (Lumbar group)

Triceps

Glutens Maximus

Biceps Femoris

Gastrocnemius

Neck

Chest Expanded

Upper Arm

Waist

Forearm

Hips

Thighs

Calf

The beginning women's program is given in recommended pounds to use, since women's weights tend to fall within a smaller range (Bill Reynolds has observed that most women in his classes weigh 100-140 lbs.). Because there is a much greater weight differential among men, it would be foolhardy to generalize poundage rates for them.

You can find the complete explanations and illustrations of each exercise referred to in the programs by turning to the alphabetical list of exercises on page 34.

If an exercise in a program doesn't agree with you — if you don't have the necessary equipment to do it properly, or if it's too easy or too hard — adjust it to suit you. You can do this by reducing the amount of weight used, or by changing the number of repetitions or sets. Or you can simply substitute another exercise that works the same muscle or muscle group.

Being able to select your own exercises will be important when you're ready to revise your program. This should be done every four to six weeks, in order to relieve yourself of possible boredom and to present new challenges to your body. Also, this permits you to work slightly different parts of your body.

Feel free to modify any of the programs (after you're suitably broken in) to suit your personal needs and ability. Be sure to train yourself hard enough (don't be too easy on yourself), yet don't overextend yourself and subject your body to injury. The important reminders at the end of this discussion will keep you on the straight and narrow path to designing a successful, personalized weight-training program.

Before you begin *any* specialized program, you should get into weight-training shape by going through one of the general fitness programs for at least four to six weeks. This will prime your muscles for the tougher workouts to come. Also, it will allow you to discover which of your muscles are weaker and need more attention.

Where advisable, an off-season, as well as an in-season, training program has been supplied for various sports. Please note that the specialized programs are listed in alphabetical order. Unless stated otherwise, they should be performed three times a week, on nonconsecutive days, e.g., Monday, Wednesday, and Friday.

Not included in the programs are the stretching exercises and such warm-up/warm-down exercises as running-in-place and jumping rope. Be sure to include several minutes of each of these kinds of activities before and after your program workout.

Some people wonder if they should complete all the sets of one exercise before moving on to the next, or if they should go through each exercise one set at a time and cycle through the entire program as many times as it takes to complete the recommended dosage of sets. The correct answer depends on what your chief goal is: general fitness (including weight reduction) or greater strength (including weight gain). If you're after general fitness, do one set of each exercise, cycle through the entire program, then go back and pick up the odd sets. If you're after strength, do all the sets of an exercise before going on the next exercise.

Important Reminders:

— Lift the amount of weight that corresponds to the correct percentage of your body weight.

— Don't be afraid to change an exercise to suit your needs and ability.

— Be clear about what your chief goal is: general fitness or greater strength. Then perform your program accordingly.

— Change your program every four to six weeks to combat boredom and to present your body with new challenges.

— Do a general fitness program before tackling a specialized one.

— Remember to always do stretching and warm-up/warm-down exercises.

— Be sure to include at least one exercise for each major body part when designing your own program.

— For purposes of improving a specific area, include two or three exercises for that area. But do not include more than eight sets for any one body part when you are still a beginning weight-trainer.

Order in Which to Exercise Body Parts:

1. Thighs
2. Back
3. Chest
4. Deltoids
5. Biceps-Triceps
6. Forearms
7. Abdominals
8. Neck, Calves

Programs include:

1. Beginning Program for Women
2. Beginning Program for Men
3. Intermediate Program for Women
4. Intermediate Program for Men
5. Archery
6. Baseball/Softball
7. Basketball
8. Bowling
9. Boxing
10. Canoeing/Kayaking
11. Crew (Rowing)
12. Cross-Country Skiing
13. Cycling
14. Dancing
15. Diving
16. Fencing
17. Football
18. Gymnastics
19. Handball
20. Ice Hockey/Field Hockey
21. Ice Skating
22. Martial Arts
23. Mountain Climbing/Hiking
24. Running (Sprinting & Long Distance/Jogging)
25. Skiing/Water Skiing
26. Soccer
27. Swimming
28. Tennis & Other Racket Sports
29. Track & Field
30. Volleyball
31. Weight Gain
32. Weight Loss
33. Wrestling

Program 1: Beginning Program for Women

Exercises	Sets	Repetitions	% of Your Body Weight
1. Clean & Press	1	10-15	20%
2. Bench Press	2	10-15	30-40%
3. Bent Arm Lateral	1	10-15	10%
4. Bentover Rowing	1	10-15	30-40%
5. Bent Arm Pullover	1	10-15	30-40%
6. Squat	2	10-15	30-40%
7. Calf Raise (Dumbbell or Barbell)	3	15-25	40-50%
8. Lunge	1	15-20	30%
9. Leg Curl	1	15	10%
10. Sit-up	1	15-30	**

**If you reach the point of being able to do fifty sit-ups easily, use a 5-lb. weight plate while doing them — and drop your number of repetitions down to twenty. Then work up to thirty, and add another 2½-5 lbs. of weight, dropping your repetitions back to twenty again.

Program 2: Beginning Program for Men

Exercises	Sets	Repetitions	% of Your Body Weight
1. Clean & Press	1	15	35%
2. Squat	3	12-15	40%
3. Bench Press	3	8-12	50%
4. Bentover Rowing	3	8-12	40%
5. Military Press	2	6-10	35%
6. Barbell Curl	2	8-12	35%
7. Calf Raise (either dumbbell or barbell)	3-5	15-25	50%
8. Stiff-Leg Deadlift	1	10-15	40%
9. Wrist Curl	1	15-20	25%
10. Sit-up	1	25-50	**

**When you reach the point of being able to do fifty sit-ups easily, use a 5 or 10-lb. weight while doing them and drop your number of repetitions down to twenty. Then work up to thirty, and add some more weight.

Program 3: Intermediate Program for Women

Exercises	Sets	Repetitions	% of Your Body Weight
1. Clean & Press	1	12-15	25%
2. Bench Squat	3	12-15	70%
3. Lunge	2	12-15	15%
4. Leg Curl	2	12-15	15%
5. Calf Raise	3	15-20	70%
6. Bentover Rowing	3	9-12	30%
7. Stiff-Leg Deadlift	1	9-12	30%
8. Bench Press	3	8-10	30%
9. Dumbbell Curl	2	8-12	20%
10. Dumbbell French Press	2	8-12	20%
11. Wrist Curl	2-3	12-20	20%
12. Sit-up	1-3	25-50	**

**When you reach the point of being able to do fifty sit-ups easily, use a 5-lb. weight plate while doing them — and drop your number of repetitions down to twenty. Work up to thirty, then add more weight and drop your repetitions back to twenty again.

Program 4: Intermediate Program for Men

Exercises	Sets	Repetitions	% of Your Body Weight
1. Clean & Press	1	12-15	35%
2. Bench Squat	3	12-15	80%
3. Leg Curl	2	12-15	20%
4. Calf Raise	3	15-20	80%
5. Bentover Rowing	3	9-12	40%
6. Shoulder Shrug	2	12-15	50%
7. Stiff-Leg Deadlift	1	9-12	40%
8. Bench Press	3-5	8-10	40%
9. Dumbbell Curl	3	8-12	30%
10. Dumbbell French Press	3	8-12	30%
11. Wrist Curl	3-5	12-20	30%
12. Sidebend	1-3	25-100	—
13. Sit-up	1-3	25-50	**

**When you reach the point of being able to do fifty sit-ups easily, use a 5-lb. weight plate while doing them — and drop your number of repetitions down to twenty-five. Work up to thirty-five, then add more weight and drop your repetitions back to twenty-five again.

Program 5: Archery

If you're weight-training primarily for the sake of improving your archery performance, you can use the following program, which concentrates on exercising your upper body. The stronger you become from weight-training, the steadier you'll be . . . and the better your aim. Upright rowing, for example, will help you to develop an abundance of pulling power. You should do this workout three times a week after shooting, and follow the same regimen whether in or out of season.

Exercises	Sets	Repetitions	Men	Women
1. Sit-up	1	25-100	—	—
2. Bench Press	2	8-12	45%	35%
3. Military Press	2	6-10	40%	30%
4. Upright Rowing	2	8-12	30%	20%
5. Reverse Curl	2	8-12	25%	15%
6. Bent Lateral	2	12-15	10%	7%
7. Dumbbell Kickback	2	12-15	20%	15%
8. Stiff-Leg Deadlift	1	10-15	40%	30%
9. Sidebend	1	15-20	—	—

Program 6: Baseball/Softball

This program will develop the muscles used in hitting and throwing. Exercises like the wrist curl will increaese hand and forearm strength, which can contribute to home-run power.

Off-Season Program (to be done three times a week, combined with a vigorous running program on alternate days):

Exercises	Sets	Repetitions	Men	Women
1. Clean & Press	1	15-20	35%	25%
2. Squat	2	12-15	50%	40%
3. Leg Curl	2	12-15	25%	15%
4. Calf Raise	3	15-25	60%	50%
5. Bench Press	2	12-15	40%	30%
6. Bentover Rowing	2	8-12	45%	35%
7. Upright Rowing	2	12-15	30%	20%
8. Press behind Neck	2	8-12	35%	25%
9. Reverse Curl	2	12-15	30%	20%
10. French Press (Dumbbell or Barbell)	2	12-15	30%	20%
11. Wrist Curl	2	20-30	20%	15%
12. Reverse Wrist Curl	2	20-30	15%	10%
13. Sit-up	1	25-100	—	—

In-Season Program (to be done twice a week, evenly spaced, e.g., Monday and Thursday, or Tuesday and Saturday, after your baseball workout or game):

1. Clean & Press	1	15-20	35%	25%
2. Squat	1	20-30	40%	30%
3. Calf Raise	2	20-30	50%	40%
4. Bench Press	1	20-30	35%	25%
5. Bentover Rowing	2	8-12	45%	35%
6. Reverse Curl	1	20-30	20%	15%
7. Wrist Curl	1	30-40	20%	10%
8. Sit-up	1	25-100	—	—

Program 7: Basketball

Basketball players often need to gain weight. To achieve this, do the exercises with heavier weights and half the number of repetitions given. Also, you can add one set to each exercise (except for abdominal ones).

Off-Season Program:

Exercises	Sets	Repetitions	Men	Women
1. Clean & Press	1	15-20	35%	25%
2. Jumping Squat	3	15-20	40%	30%
3. Lunge	2	15-20	15%	10%
4. Leg Curl	2	15-20	20%	15%
5. Calf Raise	3	20-30	60%	50%
6. Bench Press	2	12-15	40%	30%
7. Upright Rowing	1	12-15	30%	20%
8. Reverse Curl	2	12-15	30%	20%
9. Wrist Curl	2	20-30	25%	15%
10. Reverse Wrist Curl	2	20-30	15%	10%
11. Leg Raise	1	25-100	—	—

In-Season Program (to be done twice a week, evenly spaced, e.g., Monday and Thursday, or Tuesday and Saturday, after your basketball workout or game):

1. Clean & Press	1	15-20	35%	25%
2. Jumping Squat	1	15-20	40%	30%
3. Bench Press	1	12-15	40%	30%
4. Bentover Rowing	2	12-15	40%	30%
5. Side Lateral Raise	1	12-15	15%	10%
6. Reverse Curl	1	12-15	30%	20%
7. Wrist Curl	1	20-30	25%	15%
8. Leg Raise	1	25-100	—	—

Program 8: Bowling

Since bowlers can and do compete in their sport year-round, one program will suffice. Emphasis is on leg, shoulder, arm, and back strength. The program should be done three times a week after bowling practice.

Exercises	Sets	Repetitions	Men	Women
1. Squat	2	12-15	40%	30%
2. Bentover Rowing	2	8-12	40%	30%
3. Upright Rowing	1	12-15	30%	20%
4. Front Lateral Raise	2	8-12	20%	10%
5. Dumbbell Curl	1	8-12	20%	10%
6. Stiff-Leg Deadlift	2	8-15	40%	30%
7. Sit-up	1	25-100	—	—

Program 9: Boxing

There seems to be an unfounded prejudice among boxing coaches against training with weights. The myth that it will slow and tighten-up boxers is untrue. On the contrary, as for all other athletes, weight-training makes boxers more flexible, quicker, and more powerful. This program should be followed three times a week after regular boxing workouts.

Exercises	Sets	Repetitions	Men	Women
1. Jumping Rope	1	2-3 mins.	—	—
2. Jumping Squat	1	20-30	40%	30%
3. Calf Raise	2-3	15-25	60%	50%
4. Bench Press	3-4	15-20	40%	30%
5. Bentover Rowing	2	10-15	40%	30%
6. Military Press	2	10-15	35%	25%
7. Upright Rowing	2	10-15	35%	25%
8. Leg Raise	1	25-100	—	—

Program 10: Canoeing/Kayaking

This concentrates on developing torso and arm strenth, so essential for canoeing and kayaking.

Off-Season Program:

Exercises	Sets	Repetitions	Men	Women
1. Power Santch	1	12-15	50%	40%
2. Bentover Bowing	3	8-12	40%	30%
3. Upright Rowing	2	8-12	30%	20%
4. Side Lateral Raise	1	12-15	20%	10%
5. Bentover Lateral	1	12-15	20%	10%
6. Dumbbell French Press	1	12-15	20%	15%
7. Leg Press	1	15-20	20%	15%
8. Stiff-Leg Deadlift	2	8-15	50%	40%
9. Sit-up	1	15-100	—	—

As the competitive season comes up, you should shift to circuit-training. That means you should go through one set of each exercise, then repeat the entire program.

In-Season Program (to be done twice a week, evenly spaced, e.g., Monday and Thursday, or Tuesday and Saturday, after your canoeing or kayaking practice):

1. Upright Rowing	2	12-15	25%	15%
2. Bentover Rowing	2	12-15	35%	25%
3. Bent Arm Pullover	1	12-15	25%	15%
4. Squat	2	12-15	40%	30%
5. Stiff-Leg Deadlift	2	8-15	45%	35%
6. Leg Raise	2	25-50	—	—
7. Bentover Lateral	2	12-15	20%	10%

Program 11: Crew (Rowing)

Great demands are made on different muscle groups in this sport. This program is designed to increase particularly the strength of the thighs, deltoids, hamstrings, and upper and lower back.

Off-Season Program (to be done three times a week after regular crew workouts):

Exercises	Sets	Repetitions	Men	Women
1. Clean & Press	1	15-20	25%	15%
2. Squat	2	15-20	45%	35%
3. Lunge	1	15-20	20%	15%
4. Leg Curl	2	20-30	20%	10%
5. Power Clean	2	12-15	50%	40%
6. Upright Rowing	2	20-30	25%	15%
7. Bentover Rowing	2	25-35	30%	20%
8. Stiff-Leg Deadlift	1	15-20	50%	40%
9. Barbell Curl	3	15-20	30%	20%
10. Sit-up	1	50-100	—	—

As the competitive season nears, switch to circuit-training. This means doing one set of each exercise quickly, then repeating the entire program three times.

In-Season Program (to be done twice a week, evenly spaced, e.g., Monday and Thursday, or Tuesday and Saturday):

1. Upright Rowing	3	20-30	25%	15%
2. Squat	3	20-30	30%	20%
3. Power Clean	3	12-15	50%	40%
4. Sit-up	3	25-50	—	—
5. Bent Arm Pullover	3	15-20	35%	25%
6. Stiff-Leg Deadlift	3	15-20	50%	40%
7. Bentover Rowing	3	15-20	30%	20%
8. Barbell Curl	3	15-20	30%	20%
9. Leg Curl	3	20-30	20%	10%
10. Lunge	3	15-20	15%	10%
11. Good Morning	3	15-20	15%	10%

Program 12: Cross-Country Skiing

This program concentrates on leg and torso development. It should be combined with a good running program.

Off-Season Program:

Exercises	Sets	Repetitions	Men	Women
1. Squat	2-3	20-30	70%	60%
2. Jumping Squat	2	10-15	35%	25%
3. Lunge	2	20-30	20%	15%
4. Leg Curl	2	20-30	20%	15%
5. Good Morning	1	20-30	15%	10%
6. Bent Arm Pullover	3-4	12-15	40%	30%
7. Calf Raise	3-5	20-30	50%	40%
8. Sit-up	1	15-100	—	—

In-Season Program (to be done very quickly, four to six times a week):

Exercises	Sets	Repetitions	Men	Women
1. Squat	1	20-30	35%	25%
2. Leg Raise	1	30-50	—	—
3. Jumping Squat	1	12-15	35%	25%
4. Leg Curl	1	20-30	20%	10%
5. Bent Arm Pullover	1	20-30	40%	30%
6. Calf Raise	1	20-30	50%	40%
7. Good Morning	1	20-30	15%	10%
8. Sit-up	1	25-50	—	—

Program 13: Cycling

The same program can be used for off- and in-season. This program concentrates on developing thighs, hamstring and calf strength, and general endurance.

Exercises	Sets	Repetitions	Men	Women
1. Squat	2-3	20-30	45%	35%
2. Step-up	2-3	20-30	30%	20%
3. Lunge	2	15-20	25%	10%
4. Calf Raise	2-3	20-30	50%	40%
5. Seated Calf Exercise	2-3	20-30	60%	50%
6. Leg Curl	3-4	30-50	15%	10%
7. Power Clean	1	15-20	45%	35%
8. Sit-up	1	25-100	—	—
9. Wrist Curl	1-3	20-30	30%	20%

Program 14: Dancing

Although dancing isn't a sport, weight-training can be very useful for developing leg strength, flexibility, and stamina. It's no accident that dancers have bodies that are comparable to athletes in terms of superior fitness, since they have stringent, vigorous exercise programs of their own. Recently, more and more dancers have become aware of the values of weight-training for their art. This program concentrates on developing leg- and upper-body strength so that you can function more gracefully in positions in which you may have poor body mechanics.

Exercises	Sets	Repetitions	Men	Women
1. Jumping Squat	2	25-50	30%	20%
2. Lunge	2	15-20	15%	10%
3. Leg Curl	2	15-20	10%	5%
4. Good Morning	1	15-20	20%	10%
5. Bench Press	1	8-12	40%	30%
6. Bentover Rowing	1	8-12	40%	30%
7. Calf Raise	2-3	20-30	50%	40%
8. Twisting	1	25-100	—	—
9. Sidebend	1	25-100	—	—
10. Sit-up	1	25-100	—	—

Program 15: Diving

This program is designed to promote agility and flexibility, as well as strength. It emphasizes developing your legs and abdomen, and it should be done three times a week, both off- and in-season.

Exercises	Sets	Repetitions	Men	Women
1. Jumping Squat	2-3	15-20	60%	50%
2. Straddle Hop	1-2	20-30	40%	30%
3. Sit-up	1-2	30-50	—	—
4. Leg Raise	1-2	30-50	—	—
5. Knee-up	1	20-50	10%	7½%
6. Twisting	1-2	50-100	—	—

Program 16: Fencing

This program concentrates on developing legs, deltoids, biceps, and triceps. It includes exercises that can improve your fencing performance. For example, lunging strengthens your basic fencing leg movements. The bench press improves thrusting, and the wrist curl helps you parry an opponent's thrusts. Whether off- or in-season, this program should be performed three times a week.

Exercises	Sets	Repetitions	Men	Women
1. Squat	1	12-15	75%	65%
2. Lunge	2-3	12-15	35%	25%
3. Leg Curl	2-3	12-15	20%	10%
4. Upright Rowing	2	8-12	30%	20%
5. Bench Press	2	8-12	40%	30%
6. Military Press	2	8-12	30%	20%
7. Reverse Curl	2	8-12	20%	10%
8. Wrist Curl	1	20-30	25%	15%
9. Reverse Wrist Curl	2	20-30	15%	10%
10. Leg Raise	1	30-50	—	—

Program 17: Football

Studies done as far back as 1960 by the Green Bay Packers showed that football players who didn't follow weight-training maintenance program lost up to 70% of their functional strength between seasons. The programs emphasize leg and back strength, as well as chest and shoulder development.

Off-Season Program (to be done 3-4 times a week):

Exercises	Sets	Repetitions	Men	Women
1. Power Clean	3-5	6-10	50%	40%
2. Squat	3-5	8-12	80%	60%
3. Bench Press	3	8-12	50%	40%
4. Stiff-Leg Deadlift	2	12-20	40%	30%
5. Bentover Rowing	3	8-12	50%	40%
6. Military Press	2	8-12	40%	30%
7. Barbell Curl	3	8-12	35%	25%
8. Calf Raise	3-5	20-30	80%	60%
9. Seated Calf Exercise	3-5	20-30	100%	80%
10. Sidebend	1	20-50	—	—
11. Sit-up	1	20-50	—	—

In-Season Program (to be done twice a week, one and four days after a game):

1. Power Clean	2	8-12	45%	35%
2. Jumping Squat	2	10-15	60%	50%
3. Bench Press	2	8-12	45%	35%
4. Bentover Rowing	2	8-12	45%	35%
5. Military Press	2	8-12	35%	25%
6. Barbell Curl	2	8-12	30%	20%
7. Stiff-Leg Deadlift	1	10-15	35%	25%
8. Sit-up	1	25-100	—	—

Program 18: Gymnastics

There is a certain prejudice that still exists against using energy to weight-train when it comes to gymnastics. Bill Reynolds suggests that weak muscle areas be identified and specific exercises selected to improve those areas. Six to eight sets of these exercises should be done three times a week for each weak muscle group. This program is useful for the gymnast who wants a general workout:

Exercises	Sets	Repetitions	Men	Women
1. Clean & Press	1	12-15	40%	30%
2. Jumping Squat	2	12-15	50%	40%
3. Calf Raise	3-4	20-30	100%	80%
4. Upright Rowing	2	8-12	35%	25%
5. Bench Press	3	8-12	50%	40%
6. Bentover Rowing	3	8-12	50%	40%
7. Military Press	2	8-12	55%	45%
8. Front Lateral Raise	2	12-15	25%	15%
9. Barbell Curl	2	8-12	35%	25%
10. Leg Raise	1	50-100	—	—
11. Sit-up	1	50-100	—	—

Program 19: Handball

One goal here is to even out the strength in both hands. Everyone tends to favor one, so this can come in handy. This program should be done three or four times a week, spaced out evenly.

	Exercises	Sets	Repetitions	Men	Women
1.	Clean & Press	1	12-15	45%	35%
2.	Jumping Squat	2	12-15	65%	55%
3.	Lunge	2	12-15	20%	10%
4.	Leg Curl	2	15-20	20%	15%
5.	Calf Raise	2-3	20-30	50%	40%
6.	Lying Straight Arm Lateral	2	8-12	15%	10%
7.	Lying Bent Arm Lateral	2	8-12	10%	5%
8.	Side Lateral Raise	2	8-12	10%	5%
9.	Good Morning	1	8-15	15%	10%
10.	Sit-up	1	15-100	—	—

Program 20: Ice Hockey/Field Hockey

The same program can be used for both kinds of hockey, since both sports emphasize legs, arms, and shoulder strength (which are developed by this program).

	Exercises	Sets	Repetitions	Men	Women
1.	Clean & Press	1	12-15	45%	35%
2.	Power Clean	2	8-10	55%	45%
3.	Squat	2	12-15	60%	50%
4.	Leg Curl	2	12-15	20%	15%
5.	Upright Rowing	2	8-12	25%	15%
6.	Bench Press	2	8-12	50%	40%
7.	Lying Straight Arm Lateral	2	8-12	15%	10%
8.	Lying Bent Arm Lateral	2	8-12	10%	5%
9.	Side Lateral Raise	2	8-12	10%	5%
10.	Good Morning	1	8-12	15%	10%
11.	Sit-up	1	25-100	—	—
12.	Barbell Calf Raise	2-3	20-30	60%	50%

Program 21: Ice Skating

Since figure and speed skating demand mostly lower-body strength, that's what this program emphasizes. It should be done three times a week for maximum results.

Exercises	Sets	Repetitions	Men	Women
1. Bench Press	2	8-12	50%	40%
2. Bentover Rowing	2	8-12	40%	30%
3. Bench Squat	3	12-15	100%	80%
4. Front Squat	2	12-15	80%	70%
5. Lunge	1	12-15	15%	10%
6. Leg Curl	2	12-15	20%	15%
7. Good Morning	1	12-15	15%	10%
8. Seated Calf Exercise	3-5	20-30	100%	90%
9. Sidebend	1	25-100	10%	10%
10. Sit-up	1	15-100	—	—

Program 22: Martial Arts

Weight-training can be invaluable to practitioners of the martial arts, in that it can greatly increase strength and improve performance. This program is suitable for anyone involved in a martial art, as it works the entire body. This should be done three times a week.

Exercises	Sets	Repetitions	Men	Women
1. Clean & Press	1	12-15	45%	35%
2. Squat	2-3	15-20	45%	35%
3. Leg Curl	2	15-20	20%	15%
4. Stiff-Leg Deadlift	2	8-12	60%	50%
5. Bentover Rowing	3	8-12	40%	30%
6. Bench Press (Dumbbell)	3	12-15	50%	40%
7. Upright Rowing	2	8-12	40%	30%
8. Military Press	2	8-12	40%	30%
9. Dumbbell Curl (Seated)	2	8-12	35%	25%
10. Dumbbell French Press	1	12-15	20%	15%
11. Wrist Curl	2	20-30	35%	25%
12. Seated Calf Exercise	2-3	20-30	60%	50%
13. Sidebend	1	25-100	10%	10%
14. Twisting	1	25-100	10%	10%
15. Sit-up	1	25-100	—	—

Program 23: Mountain Climbing/Hiking

Mountain climbing and hiking make demands on your entire body, with speical emphasis on your legs. This program helps develop strength in all ares, especially legs. Year-round, this program can be performed three times a week.

Exercises	Sets	Repetitions	Men	Women
1. Clean & Press	1	12-15	45%	35%
2. Shoulder Shrug	3	12-15	60%	50%
3. Bentover Rowing	3	8-12	40%	30%
4. Stiff-Leg Deadlift	1-2	8-12	40%	30%
5. Bench Press	3	8-12	60%	40%
6. Bent Arm Pullover	2-3	12-15	40%	30%
7. Step-up	3	15-20	50%	40%
8. Squat	2-3	15-20	45%	35%
9. Calf Raise	2-3	20-30	50%	40%
10. Reverse Curl	2	12-15	25%	15%
11. Wrist Curl	2	20-30	40%	30%
12. Knee-up	1	20-30	—	—

Program 24: Running

Sprinting (for people running 100-400 meters, this program develops the powerful leg drive necessary for sprinting):

1. Clean &

Exercises	Sets	Repetitions	Men	Women
1. Clean & Press	1-2	12-15	45%	35%
2. Squat	2-3	12-15	45%	35%
3. Leg Extension	2-3	12-15	20%	15%
4. Leg Curl	2	12-15	20%	15%
5. Calf Raise	3-5	20-30	50%	40%
6. Bench Press	2-3	8-12	50%	40%
7. Bentover Rowing	2-3	8-12	40%	30%
8. Upright Rowing	2-3	8-12	40%	30%
9. Sit-up	1	25-100	—	—
10. Good Morning	1	15-20	—	—

Distance/Jogging (for people who run longer distances, this program develops those muscles that don't receive a sufficient workout from running. For example, a runner's quadriceps usually are underdeveloped in relation to his or her hamstrings; this results in knee imbalance and subjects the runner to pain and possible injury):

Exercises	Sets	Repetitions	Men	Women
1. Clean & Press	1	15-20	45%	35%
2. Bench Squat	1-2	20-30	100%	80%
3. Leg Extension	1-2	20-30	20%	15%
4. Leg Curl	1	20-30	20%	15%
5. Upright Rowing	1-2	10-15	40%	30%
6. Military Press	1-2	10-15	40%	30%
7. Sit-up	1-2	25-100	—	—

Program 25: Skiing/Water Skiing

Both types of skiing (snow/alpine and water) call on strength from your thighs and upper body. Bill Reynolds says that weekend athletes who injure themselves at the end of the day because of fatigue can benefit from this conditioning program. And all alpine ski and water ski enthusiasts can improve their performance in these sports.

Exercises	Sets	Repetitions	Men	Women
1. Squat	2-3	15-20	45%	35%
2. Lunge	2	12-15	15%	10%
3. Leg Curl	3	15-20	20%	15%
4. Calf Raise	2-3	20-30	50%	40%
5. Bench Press	3	15-20	45%	35%
6. Bentover Rowing	3	12-15	45%	35%
7. Wrist Curl	3	15-20	40%	30%
8. Good Morning	1	10-15	15%	10%
9. Sit-up	1-2	50-100	—	—
10. Leg Raise	1-2	50-100	—	—

Program 26: Soccer

This program will work for both in- and off-season training. It concentrates on developing leg muscles — enhancing quickness and strength, which are key to soccer.

Exercises	Sets	Repetitions	Men	Women
1. Clean & Press	1	12-15	40%	30%
2. Squat	2	15-20	45%	35%
3. Lunge	2	12-15	15%	10%
4. Leg Curl	1	15-20	20%	15%
5. Calf Raise	2-3	20-30	50%	40%
6. Bent Arm Pullover	1	8-12	40%	30%
7. French Press (Dumbbell or Barbell)	1	8-12	25%	15%
8. Sidebend	1	25-100	10%	10%
9. Sit-up	1	25-100		

Program 27: Swimming

Weight-training is very popular among champion swimmers and their coaches. The East Germans have demonstrated the positive results of this type of training or swimming.

Exercises	Sets	Repetitions	Men	Women
1. Squat	2-3	15-20	50%	40%
2. Leg Curl	2-3	20-30	30%	20%
3. Good Morning	1	12-15	15%	10%
4. Bentover Rowing	3	8-12	40%	30%
5. Bent Arm Pullover	3-5	15-20	50%	40%
6. Straight Arm Pullover	3-4	15-20	20%	15%
7. Leg Raise	1-3	15-20	—	—
8. Sit-up	1-3	25-100	—	—

Program 28: Tennis & Other Racket Sports (Squash, Badminton, Racquetball)

All these racket sports emphasize leg, torso and arm strength. This program exercises those body parts in particular, and aims at developing extra strength that can significantly increase your power and overall performance in these sports. The wrist and reverse curl develop strength in your hands and forearms so that you can hold the racket firmly while volleying or returning a serve. The bent lateral is key for increasing backhand strength. The French press is a key movement for preventing tennis elbow.

Exercises	Sets	Repetitions	Men	Women
1. Power Snatch	1	12-15	40%	30%
2. Bench Squat	3	15-20	90%	80%
3. Lunge	2	12-15	15%	10%
4. Leg Curl	2	12-15	30%	15%
5. Good Morning	1	12-15	15%	10%
6. Lying Straight Arm Lateral	2	8-12	30%	20%
7. Lying Bent Arm Lateral	2	8-12	15%	10%
8. Front Lateral Raise	2	8-12	15%	10%
9. Side Lateral Raise	2	8-12	15%	10%
10. Reverse Curl (Barbell)	2	8-12	30%	20%
11. French Press	2	8-12	35%	25%
12. Wrist Curl	3	15-20	40%	30%
13. Reverse Wrist Curl	3	15-20	20%	15%
14. Calf Riase	2-3	20-30	50%	40%
15. Sit-up or Leg Raise	1	25-100	—	—

Program 29: Track & Field

This is a general program for all track and field events. It should be done three times a week. For specific, advanced programs for individual events, you should consult Bill Reynold's *Complete Weight Training.*

Exercises	Sets	Repetitions	Men	Women
1. Squat	2-3	15-20	45%	35%
2. Bench Press	3-4	8-12	50%	40%
3. Bentover Rowing	3-4	8-12	45%	35%
4. Stiff-Leg Deadlift	2-3	8-12	60%	50%
5. Upright Rowing	2-3	8-12	35%	25%
6. Military Press	3	6-10	40%	30%
7. Barbell Curl	3	8-12	35%	25%
8. Wrist Curl	3	15-20	35%	25%
9. Sit-up	1-3	25-100	—	—

Program 30: Volleyball

Weight-training (especially the jumping squat) can dramatically improve a volleyball player's vertical jumping ability — very important to this sport. Bill Reynolds maintains that an increase of six inches is plausible within two to three months if a weight-training program is followed faithfully. This program is appropriate for both in- and off-season training:

Exercises	Sets	Repetitions	Men	Women
1. Clean & Press	1	12-15	40%	30%
2. Jumping Squat	2-3	12-15	60%	50%
3. Bench Squat	2-3	12-15	100%	80%
4. Calf Raise	2-3	20-30	50%	40%
5. Straddle Hop	3-5	20-30	50%	40%
6. Bentover Rowing	2-3	12-15	45%	35%
7. Bent Arm Pullover	2-3	12-15	50%	40%
8. Military Press	2-3	6-10	40%	30%
9. Good Morning	1	15-20	15%	10%
10. Sit-up	1	25-100	—	—

Program 31: Weight Gain

The idea of this program is to include basic exercise that can be performed with very heavy weights, low repetitions, and a high number of sets.

Important Points to Remember:

— Try to increase the weight on each set of a given exercise, so that by the final set you are using your maximum (this is why extreme percentages of your body weight are given).

— Avoid doing more than one set of abdominal exercises per workout (this will slow down your weight gain).

— To increase muscle mass and size, it is necessary to increase the amount of weight you lift. So, as often as possible, add poundage.

Exercises	Sets	Repetitions	Men	Women
1. Squat	1	15	30%	20%
2. (Repeat) Squat	5	6-8	50-100%	50-100%
3. Bench Press	1	15	20%	15%
4. (Repeat) Bench Press	5	4-6	40-100%	40-100%
5. Bentover Rowing	1	15	25%	15%
6. (Repeat) Bentover Row	5	6-8	40-100%	40-100%
7. Bent Arm Pullover	3	12-15	40-60%	40-60%
8. Press behind Neck	2	6-8	30-45%	25-45%
9. Barbell Curl	3	6-8	30-45%	25-45%

10. Shoulder Shrug	3	10-15	60-100%	50-100%
11. Stiff-Leg Deadlift	1	10-15	60-100%	50-100%
12. Sit-up	1	15-20	—	—
13. Calf Raise	3-5	15-20	60-100%	50-100%

Program 32: Weight Loss

In addition to helping you lose weight, this is a fine program for general conditioning and aerobic fitness. It's a toughie, so be sure to break yourself in by doing a general fitness program for at least four weeks. Because you are to perform four separate series of exercises quickly, you may find it necessary to do this particular program at a gym or spa (where there are handy fixed weights) . . . or, if you can afford it, buy additional equipment to use at home (so you won't have to spend as much time changing weights).

Important Points to Remember:

— Do each series twice before going on to the next one.

— Keep repetitions in all exercises within the 8-15 range.

— Average one set per 45-60 seconds of exercise time. You should be able to do forty total sets within 30-40 minutes. Go through these exercises rapidly. Try to achieve a breathless state throughout the workout.

Series I

Exercises	Sets	Repetitions	Men	Women
1. Squat	2	8-15	30%	20%
2. Sit-up	2	8-15	—	—
3. Bench Press	2	8-15	20%	15%
4. Wrist Curl	2	8-15	35%	25%
5. Bentover Rowing	2	8-15	25%	15%

Series II

1. Press behind Neck	2	8-15	35%	25%
2. Leg Curl	2	8-15	30%	20%
3. Lying Straight Arm Lateral	2	8-15	15%	10%
4. Twisting	2	8-15	—	—
5. Bentover Rowing (Dumbbell)	2	8-15	25%	15%

Series III

1. Stiff-Leg Deadlift	2	8-15	60%	50%
2. Shoulder Shrug	2	8-15	60%	50%
3. Barbell Curl	2	8-15	35%	25%
4. Sidebend	2	8-15	10%	10%
5. Calf Raise	2	8-15	50%	40%

Series IV

1. Upright Rowing	2	8-15	40%	30%
2. Seated Calf Exercise	2	8-15	100%	90%
3. Dumbbell Curl	2	8-15	20%	10%
4. Leg Raise	2	8-15	—	—
5. Bent Arm Pullover	2	8-15	40%	30%

Program 33: Wrestling

This program addresses itself to developing overall body strength, with particular attention given to neck, chest, shoulders, and upper back. Strength in these areas is especially needed in wrestling.

Off-Season Program:

	Exercises	Sets	Repetitions	Men
1.	Power Snatch	2-3	6-8	45%
2.	Jumping Squat	3-4	12-15	60%
3.	Bench Press	3-5	8-12	75%
4.	Upright Rowing	3	8-12	45%
5.	Military Press	3	6-10	50%
6.	Bentover Rowing (Dumbbell)	3	8-12	60%
7.	Shoulder Shrug	3	15-20	90%
8.	Good Morning	2-3	15-20	30%
9.	Barbell Curl	3-5	8-12	45%
10.	Wrist Curl	3-5	15-20	40%
11.	Leg Raise	3	15-20	—

In-Season Program (to be done twice a week, evenly spaced, e.g., Monday and Thrusday, or Tuesday and Saturday):

1.	Clean & Press	1	8-12	60%
2.	Squat	2-3	15-20	45%
3.	Bench Press	2	8-12	75%
4.	Shoulder Shrug	1	15-20	90%
5.	Bent Arm Pullover	1	10-12	50%
6.	Good Morning	1	15-20	35%
7.	Barbell Curl	1	8-12	45%
8.	Military Press	1	6-10	50%
9.	Leg Raise	1	30-50	—

5
Self-Evaluation

Lift for Life

There are many ways to keep track of your progress. One, as I said earlier, is to check in with your body in a mirror from time to time. You can also take photographs of yourself, say once a month, and keep a pictorial journal of the results of your weight-training.

Another, more objective approach, is to measure yourself at the beginning and conclusion of each program (once every four-six weeks). You should keep in mind, however, that when You're a beginner at weight-training you will make the biggest gains in girth. After you've been training for a while, you may wish to space out your self-measurements to allow more time for changes in your size.

Before beginning your first weight-training program, record your measurements. If you want to be really accurate, have someone else do the measuring. Always take your measurements *before* you exercise (not after you pump up). Use a tape measure wrapped snugly — don't force it too tight — around the part of your body to be measured.

Be sure to measure the corresponding parts of arms and legs on both sides of your body. That way you can find out if you should be doing more dumbbell or iron boot exercises to even out the strength (and size) of your two sides.

Generally, you should measure the various body parts where they are the widest (see illustration). Parts you'll probably want to measure include:

—Neck
—Chest
—Upper Arms
—Forearms
—Waist
—Hips
—Thighs
—Calves

You may also wish to measure your wrists, ankles, and knees. Use Chart A (page 000) to keep track of your "latest developments."

It's probably a good idea to log your program progress as well. Chart B (page 000) has been provided to help you do this. (You might want to photocopy it so that you'll have enough blank charts to last you for a while.)

Is There No End?

If you're already wondering when you can stop training, relax. You can stop anytime you like. In fact, you *should* take a breather every once in a while. How frequently you should have day off or a layoff period (a week) depends on your motivation, how hard you're training, and how bored or tired you've become.

But if you're harboring secret thoughts of dropping out of weight-training as soon as you get your body where you want it to be, you're in for some rethinking. If you do cease to train and do not replace it with a physically active program of comparable vigor, you can expect to slowly regress to the condition you were in before you started weight-training.

Like getting older, this is a difficult thing for some people to deal with. If you reach a point where you really like what you and your body have accomplished, and you simply want to maintain that appearance, instead of continuing to increase your poundages you can follow (indefinitely) the same program. Still, you will probably want to increase your poundages after a while, because the workout will become too easy for you, and you'll get bored. Also, your muscles will crave some progression.

As Evelyn Hsu reminds her students, "You have to continue for the rest of your life if that's the way you want to look. If you don't, you'll gradually start to flab out again. You've got to keep going with it. That's the hardest thing, I know . . . But you have to accept that your whole life changes, and that weight-training becomes an ongoing thing."

Lifting for Life

I hope this book has encouraged you to tackle weight-training. If you've been reading carefully, you'll realize my intentions are hardly diabolical. The idea is simply to get people back into their bodies, so they can function more creatively, clearly, energetically, and happily. So that all of us — no matter where we're coming from or going — can look at ourselves in the mirror and delight in what we see.

I like the way that "athletic chaplain" Robert Abraham Zuver says it: "If you're going to have to live in the machine very long . . . you should try to take reasonably good care of it, or it'll treat you like a dog, and you'll feel like a dog while you're in there. The secret in life . . . in mental, physical, and spiritual happiness and balance . . . is spelled in one word. It's the one word·the American public has never learned to spell, and that's 'moderation.' If they could learn to spell it, of course, we'd have life made."

Not being as pessimistic as Zuver, I have great confidence in everyone's ability to spell. I think if you only give weight-training a try, you'll get wonderfully hooked on it. And you'll happily continue to lift . . . for your health, strength, spirit, and for life.

6
Sources

If this book has succeeded in getting you revved up to weight-train, you may wish additional information — both practical and academic. In the end there's nothing like good, personal instruction, which you can get from professional instructors, athletic coaches, athletes who have experimented with different programs, and other people who are simply more experienced in weight-training. You can easily tell if someone is an advanced weight-trainer; he or she will exude an enviable air of confidence in the weight room and will move surely and gracefully from exercise to exercise.

With weight-training becoming a hot media item, there are many new books in the works. And every magazine you pick up seems to mention something about the growing passion for physical fitness, including lifting weights.

If you want to read just one other book or if you're seriously interested in becoming a bona fide bodybuilder, I strongly recommend Bill Reynold's comprehensive book *Complete Weight Training.* It was originally published in 1976 by World Publications (P.O. Box 366, Mountain View, California 94040). It's a hardback book and sells for $6.95.

Other books that might be helpful, intriguing, or just plain fun:

Columbu, Franco, with George Fels. *Winning Bodybuilding.* Chicago: Henry Regnery Company, 1977. Includes programs and advice for beginning, intermediate, and advanced bodybuilders. Lots of photos of the remarkable Columbu going through his exercises. (Paperback)

Fallon, Michael, and Saunders, Jim. *Muscle Building.* New York: Arco Books, various editions. Primarily for men interested in bodybuilding and increasing muscle mass. Includes line drawings and photos.

Franz, Edward. *Beginning Weight Training.* Belmont, California: Wadsworth Publishing Company, Inc., 1969. Good basic guide, with line drawings. (Paperback)

Gaines, Charles, and Butler, George. *Pumping Iron.* New York: Simon and Schuster, 1974. A fascinating introduction to the world of bodybuilding, interestingly written and artfully photographed. Terrific for rounding out one's perspective on the ultimate goal of weight-training. (Paperback)

Heidenstam, Oscar. *Modern Bodybuilding.* Buchanan, New York: Emerson Books, Inc. Revised edition. A complete guide to bodybuilding and fitness by an Englishman who really knows his stuff. A multitude of line drawings and some photos.

Hoffman, Bob. *Weight Training for Athletes.* New York: The Ronald Press Company, 1961. Exercises and programs and how they relate to different sports. Comprehensive how-to instructions with photos.

Murray, Jim, and Karpovich, Peter V. *Weight Training in Athletics.* Englewood Cliffs, New Jersey: Prentice-Hall, 1956. An older, slightly antiquated approach to weight-training and sports. Includes some good, basic advice, as well as both photos and drawings.

Randall, Bruce. *The Barbell Way to Physical Fitness.* New York: Doubleday, 1970. Written by a former Mr. Universe, this is a book full of photographs and advice about the use of barbells and weight-training.

Ravelle, Lou. *Bodybuilding for Everyone.* Buchanan, New York: Emerson Books, 1965. A general, introductory book for anyone interested in improving appearance or fitness. Includes both drawings and photos.

There are many bodybuilding magazines that can be found on newsstands. For the average weight-trainer, they may not all be helpful, but here are some likely to be of more general interest:

Iron Man (bimonthly). Iron Man Publishing Company, 512 Black Hills Avenue, Alliance, Nebraska 69301.

Muscle Mag International (quarterly). Health Culture, 270 Rutherford Road South, Brampton, Ontario, Canada L6W 3K7.

Muscular Development (bimonthly). Muscle Man, Inc., 1664 Utica Avenue, Brooklyn, New York 11234.

Strength & Health (bimonthly). Strength & Health, P.O. Box 1707, York, Pennsylvania 17405.

Also, I heartily recommend two very entertaining, informative, and sensitive films on the phenomenon and reality of bodybuilding: *Stay Hungry,* starring Jeff Bridges, Sally Field, and Arnold Scwarzenegger. Directed by Bob Rafelson and based on the book by Charles Gaines, this was a "small" film, very nicely acted and produced. A fictional side of what it's like in the world of bodybuilding. Then, of course, there's the movie version of *Pumping Iron,* also by Gaines, with George Butler. It includes all the current bodybuilding champions and succeeds in being a rather unique and entertaining documentary. Also, it will probably teach you something about how to look at your own body . . . .

Chart A

LATEST DEVELOPMENTS

Date																				
Neck																				
Chest																				
Rt. Upper Arm																				
Left Upper Arm																				
Rt. Forearm																				
Left Forearm																				
Waist																				
Hips																				
Rt. Thigh																				
Left Thigh																				
Rt. Calf																				
Left Calf																				

Chart B

PROGRAM PROGRESS

Exercise

	Poundage	Sets	Repetitions	Poundage	Sets	Repetitions	Poundage	Sets	Repetitions	Poundage	Sets	Repetitions	Poundage	Sets	Repetitions	Poundage	Sets	Repetitions	Poundage	Sets	Repetitions	Poundage	Sets	Repetitions
Date																								
Date																								
Date																								
Date																								
Date																								
Date																								
Date																								
Date																								
Date																								
Date																								
Date																								
Date																								
Date																								
Date																								

Notes

Chapter 1: Introduction

1. Geng, "Muscle Over Mind"
2. Columbu, *Winning Bodybuilding*
3. Nyad, "Pumping Iron," *womenSports*
4. King, "Publisher's Letter," *womenSports*
5. Rasch, *Weight Training*
6. Johnson, "A Little Weightlifting to Get into Feminine Shape"
7. *Ibid.*
8. Koslow, "Why Do Women Want to be Jocks?"
9. Nyad, "Pumping Iron"
10. *Ibid.*
11. Cohn, "Pumping Chic: The Launching of a New Folk Hero"
12. Murray, *Weight Lifting*
13. Johnson, "A Little Weightlifting to Get into Feminine Shape"
14. Koslow, "Why Do Women Want to be Jocks?"
15. Geng, "Muscle Over Mind"
16. Hoffman, *Weight Training for Athletes*
17. Murray & Karpovich, *Weight Training in Athletics*
18. *Ibid.*

Chapter 2: Determining Your Personal Goals

1. Hoffman, *Weight Training for Athletes*
2. Gaines & Butler, *Pumping Iron*
3. McManus, "Doing It for God and the Fat Lady"

Chapter 3: Doing It

1. Rasch, *Weight Training*
2. Hoffman, *Weight Training for Athletes*
3. Columbu, *Winning Bodybuilding*
4. Gaines & Butler, *Pumping Iron*
5. Columbu, *Winning Bodybuilding*
6. Rasch, *Weight Training*
7. Gaines & Butler, *Pumping Iron*
8. Murray & Karpovich, *Weight Training in Athletics*
9. Dellinger, "Barbell-Dumbbell Training Course"

Bibliography

—— Cohn, Nik. "Pumping Chic: The Launching of a New Folk Hero," *New York,* January 24, 1977.

—— Columbu, Franco, with George Fels. *Winning Bodybuilding.* Chicago: Henry Regnery Company, 1977.

—— Dellinger, Jack. "Barbell-Dumbbell Training Course." (Pamphlet)

—— Gaines, Charles, and Butler, George. *Pumping Iron.* New York: Simon and Schuster, 1974.

—— Geng, Veronica. "Muscle Over Mind," *Ms.,* October 1975.

—— Hoffman, Bob. *Weight Training for Athletes.* New York: The Ronald Press Company, 1961.

—— Johnson, Sharon. "A Little Weightlifting to Get into Feminine Shape," *New York Times,* September 13, 1976.

—— King, Billy Jean. "Publisher's Letter," *womenSports,* April 1977.

—— Koslow, Sally Platkin. "Why Do Women Want to be Jocks?" *Mademoiselle,* August 1975.

—— McManus, Kathy. "Doing It for God and the Fat Lady," *new magazine* (no date).

—— Murray, Jim. *Weight Lifting.* London: Thorsons Publishers, Ltd., 1955.

—— Murray, Jim. and Peter V. Karpovich, M.D. *Weight Training in Athletics.* Englewood Cliffs, New Jersey: Prentice-Hall, Inc., 1956.

—— Nyad, Diana. "Pumping Iron," *womenSports,* April 1977.

—— Rasch, Philip. *Weight Training.* Dubuque, Iowa: Wm. C. Brown Company Publishers, 1975 (Second Edition).

—— Reynolds, Bill. *Complete Weight Training Book.* Mountian View, California: World Publications, 1976.

—— Tym, Alice. "Weight Training for the Tennis Player," *World Tennis,* December 1976.